SUPER FOODS
SUPER LIFE

Madhur Kotharay holds a BTech degree from IIT Bombay and an MS in Solid State Physics from Princeton University in the United States. In 1991, he returned to India to launch Analgesia, which became India's leading medical software brand. He created and launched computer training courses designed specifically for doctors, in biostatistics, telemedicine and computer-based medical diagnosis. Kotharay began creating medical content in 1997, after discovering the gaps in India's medical systems and becoming convinced of the importance of preventive medicine. Since then, he has written articles and blogs on preventive healthcare. He has run full marathons every year since 1989, totalling 188, including fifty-two in 2011, a national record at the time.

Advance Praise for *Superfoods, Super Life*

'Well-researched ... unravels the myriad health benefits of these foods in an engaging and easy-to-read manner. The book highlights that while no single food is a panacea for all your health challenges, it can be your ally in achieving optimal health. This perspective is crucial in a world where food trends and simplistic health solutions often overshadow the complexities of health and wellness'

Dr Shabnam Das Kar, MD, FMNM, functional medicine doctor and brain health coach

'Madhur Kotharay's medical knowledge and reasoning, which surpasses that of many practitioners, is astounding ... His greatest strength is his ability to understand and explain the differences between preventive and curative medicine more effectively than most'

Dr Girish Dani, MD, FCPS, DGO, DFP, obstetrician and gynaecologist

'This book will encourage everyone to learn more about how twenty simple ingredients can help achieve improved health. Madhur Kotharay has made this task very simple'

Dr Lily Kiswani, MD, DGO, gynaecologist, integrative medicine specialist and India's first female laparoscopic surgeon

'Redefines healing through nutritionally dense foods ... *Superfoods, Super Life* is a gift to mankind, especially for those looking for healing through foods. This book marks a major step forward from preventive to regenerative medicine'

Dr Rajshree Vachhrajani, MS and PhD, nutritional science, nutritional medicine specialist and Founder, Ultra Wellness

SUPER FOODS SUPER LIFE

20 INDIAN INGREDIENTS
to Prevent Disease and
Uplift Your Health

MADHUR KOTHARAY

PAN

First published 2024 by Pan
an imprint of Pan Macmillan Publishing India Private Limited
707 Kailash Building
26 K. G. Marg, New Delhi 110001
www.panmacmillan.co.in

Pan Macmillan, The Smithson, 6 Briset Street, Farringdon, London EC1M 5NR
Associated companies throughout the world
www.panmacmillan.com

ISBN 978-93-95624-85-5

Copyright © Madhur Kotharay 2024

The moral rights of the author have been asserted.

The views expressed in this book are the author's own and the facts reported
by him have been verified by the publisher to the extent possible.
The publisher hereby disclaims any liability to any party for loss,
damages or disruptions caused by the same.

All rights reserved. No part of this publication may be reproduced, stored
in or introduced into a retrieval system, or transmitted, in any form, or by
any means (electronic, mechanical, photocopying, recording or otherwise)
without the prior written permission of the publisher. Any person who does
any unauthorized act in relation to this publication may be liable to criminal
prosecution and civil claims for damages.

1 3 5 7 9 8 6 4 2

This book is sold subject to the condition that it shall not, by way of trade
or otherwise, be lent, re-sold, hired out, or otherwise circulated without the
publisher's prior consent in any form of binding or cover other than that in
which it is published and without a similar condition including this condition
being imposed on the subsequent purchaser.

Typeset in Minion Pro by R. Ajith Kumar, New Delhi
Printed and bound in India by Thomson Press India Ltd.

For the thousands of well-wishers who trusted my health advice over the last thirty years

CONTENTS

Introduction — xi

1. Tomato — 1
   Antioxidant Elixir

2. Garlic — 16
   Heart Guardian

3. Cinnamon — 33
   Diabetes Warrior

4. Green Tea — 49
   Modern-day Sanjivani

5. Papaya — 72
   Platelet Regulator

6. Spinach — 87
   Eye and Skin Guard

7. Ginger — 104
   Digestive Dynamo

8. Aloe Vera — 118
   Skin Health Expert

9. Turmeric — 134
   Liver Protector

10. Carrot 152
Eye Specialist

11. Flaxseed 173
Omega-3 Powerhouse

12. Amla (Indian Gooseberry) 188
Immunity Superstar

13. Pineapple 202
Joint-Protective Sentinel

14. Coconut 218
Hair Specialist

15. Jamun (Java Plum) 235
Diabetes Defender

16. Capsicum (Bell Peppers) 247
Heart Protector

17. Asafoetida (Hing) 257
Digestive Powerhouse

18. Moringa (Drumsticks) 271
Antioxidant All-Rounder

19. Sabja (Sweet Basil Seeds) 286
Fibre Friend

20. Beetroot 299
Endurance Booster

Appendix A: When is a Food Item a Good Nutrient Source? 313
Appendix B: Summary of Health Benefits from Nutrients 326
Appendix C: Overview of Nutrients in Food Items 328
Notes and References 330

INTRODUCTION

An elderly gentleman was searching for something on the floor of a bar. When asked what he was looking for, he said, 'My car keys.' Soon, a couple of well-intentioned Samaritans joined the hunt. After a few fruitless minutes, a young man enquired, 'Where exactly did you drop the keys?' The older man directed his finger to a dimly lit corner of the cavernous bar and replied, 'There.' Exasperated, the young man asked, 'Then why are you searching for them here?'

Unruffled, he responded, 'Because it is too dark over there.'

While we may share a chuckle over this anecdote, it mirrors our approach to seeking health through food. We tend to look for answers in the usual spots, yet the true keys to well-being lie elsewhere. This book aims to shine a light on obscure corners of the nutrition world, where the secrets to good health can be discovered. Let me explain further.

You've likely heard of the concept 'we are what we eat'. Many of the foods we consume are loaded with nutrients that support our health. Carrots, tomatoes, beets, spinach and many others are rightly called superfoods – nature's own medicines. This book explores how they can enhance our overall wellness.

To do this, I reviewed over ten thousand scientific papers and abstracts on their health effects, narrowing it down to 1,600 references. Thus, the book you hold is rooted in scientific evidence, not anecdotal experiences, providing a comprehensive understanding of the power of superfoods.

When it comes to seeking wellness through nutritious foods, however, we make four major mistakes, looking for the keys to our health in the wrong places simply because they are bright and conspicuous.

1. We focus on the wrong nutrients in our foods.

When I first started researching the vitamins and minerals in our superfoods, I wanted to give straightforward advice like, 'Carrots are rich in vitamin A, which helps prevent dry, scaly and itchy skin', or 'Spinach, with its magnesium, helps prevent muscle cramps and fatigue'.

But as I pored over research papers, I found at best a couple of paragraphs discussing the role of vitamins and minerals in our superfoods; they seemed less significant than anticipated. The papers often concluded that the benefits stemmed from compounds with complicated, lesser-known names, like betalains, kaempferol, chymopapain and umbelliprenin. Who has even heard of them?

The result was stark: 95 per cent of the book's planned content became irrelevant. The true heroes within superfoods turned out to be different from the ones I had initially sought.

With over thirty years of experience with the medical field, twenty-four of which were dedicated to preventive healthcare, I am far from a novice. Yet, the magnitude of the gap between what we perceive to be important and what is actually significant astounded me.

Of course, our superfoods are packed with vitamins and minerals essential for the efficient and optimum functioning of our bodies. But if that is your sole focus, then a high-quality multivitamin, multimineral supplement could be a simpler solution. Just make sure it's plant-based for better benefits, thus allowing you to sidestep the entire hustle and bustle surrounding fruits and vegetables.

For example, you don't need to specifically eat bell peppers to get vitamin B_6, which can also be obtained from other sources like amla (Indian gooseberry), spinach or a vitamin supplement. However, bromelain, a super-nutrient that improves joint health, is found exclusively in pineapple – no other edible sources exist worldwide. So, consuming moringa leaves for vitamin B_6 is not a health hack, but drinking pineapple juice for healthier joints may be.

To be sure, we won't ignore the vitamin and mineral contents of our superfoods: appendix C contains detailed information on the amounts found in various foods. Individual chapters also highlight the vitamins and minerals that each food contains. Nonetheless, the focus of this book is primarily on these complex-sounding super-nutrients.

2. We expect these superfoods to alleviate the wrong set of ailments.

We tend to link food to nutrients that ward off minor issues such as fatigue, hair fall, dull skin, cold, cough, heartburn, muscle cramps, constipation or weight gain. But these superfoods can help alleviate more serious conditions, such as diabetes, heart disease, dementia, fatty liver, arthritis and different types of cancers. To delve deeper into which superfoods can counter these degenerative diseases, refer to appendix B.

3. Our incorrect understanding of diseases stemming from heart, liver, brain, bone and joint disorders fails to prevent their onset.

As I continued reading studies, a recurring pattern emerged: each healthy food worked against multiple 'categories' of diseases. Why would an ingredient that prevents eye disorders also protect against heart disease? Why would a superfood that helps manage diabetes also ward off joint damage? It seemed that these disorders treated by various 'medical specialties' were similar diseases manifesting in different organs.

Imagine two mobile phones positioned on the edge of a table. A minor jolt to the table causes them to fall to the ground, cracking the display of one and breaking the camera lens of the other. The two issues stemming from the same incident lead to different consequences. Moving the phones to the centre of the table could have prevented them from getting damaged.

Many degenerative disorders arise in a similar manner: some mechanisms cause a few cells to malfunction. Depending on where they are located, problems start manifesting in that system, triggering distress in more cells and resulting in a cascading effect that leads to disease in that organ.

These disorders manifest in different organs, depending on which body cells are affected: brain inflammation (dementia or Parkinson's disease), insulin resistance in muscle cells (diabetes), LDL cholesterol oxidation in heart arteries (heart disease), bone mass thinning (fragile bones or osteoporosis) or joint cartilage deterioration (osteoarthritis). A weakened immune system allows uncontrolled cell growth (cancer) in some people, while an overactive immune system attacks the body itself (autoimmune conditions like rheumatoid arthritis or psoriasis) in others.

I came across the names of the culprits again and again: 'oxidative stress', the scientific term for these destructive forces, and 'inflammation', the toxic environment created as the body's response to distress.

Why is this important? Let's go back to the example of the two mobile phones. The solution there was to shift the phones to the centre of the table. But once the screens had cracked, both phones needed different treatments: one required display change, the other a lens replacement.

Similarly, preventing heart disease, dementia or osteoarthritis necessitates the same solution: reducing oxidative stress and inflammation. But once afflicted with one of the conditions, your treatment options diverge: a cardiologist for heart disease, a neurophysician for memory loss and an orthopaedic surgeon for osteoarthritis.

Our superfoods are prevention experts, reducing oxidative stress and inflammation. While each nutrient works differently, the end result is the same: to combat the two adversaries of your health. No wonder then that most superfoods protect against multiple degenerative diseases, as you will read in the book.

In other words, to prevent diseases, they need to be first attributed to the right causes. For example, if we consider fragile bones a consequence of low bone calcium and rely on calcium-rich foods, they may not prevent the problem. Osteoporosis is set off by oxidative stress, followed by inflammation. By integrating anti-inflammatory foods like bell peppers, tomatoes, garlic, ginger and green tea – all of which are poor calcium sources – into our diet, we can better protect our bone health.

But can our superfoods help once we are afflicted with a disease? Many lifestyle diseases are progressive in nature. Diabetes, high blood pressure, cancers and eczema don't go away on their own. Even with treatment, rheumatoid arthritis and Parkinson's disease worsen with time. This is partly because the kindling flames also stoke the fire when it erupts. Oxidative stress and inflammation make dementia, fatty liver and heart disease progressively severe.

Our superfoods can prevent these two enemies from adding fuel to the fire. Smaller fires will fall under control, allowing us to attribute curative properties to our superfoods.

Yet, some infernos will spiral out of control, needing medical treatment far beyond the capabilities of our foods, which brings me to our fourth misconception.

4. We expect our foods to work like medicines.

When it comes to diseases like diabetes, high blood pressure, and an underactive thyroid, we frequently rely on medication. While these medicines provide immediate relief, they do not provide a long-term cure. Similarly, we expect our foods to offer the same quick solution.

But superfoods work over time, addressing the underlying causes of oxidative damage and degenerative inflammation. For example, if you become ill and are unable to cook, you may order food from nearby food joints as a stop-gap arrangement. But relying on restaurant food for an extended period of time may not be healthy or meet your taste preferences. The long-term solution is to get your health back on track; however, without the takeaway food, you would go hungry in the short term. Both measures play an important role in their respective time frames.

Medicines are like restaurant food because they do the job your body cannot at a certain point. If your arteries can't lower your blood pressure, medicines try to slow down your heart (beta-blockers) or reduce water in your blood (diuretics). They work fast and do their job well. But they don't fix the problem and, like outside food, they can have side effects.

Superfoods work differently. They slowly repair your body, by lowering insulin resistance in diabetes and making blood vessels less rigid in a high blood pressure condition, for instance. When you're sick, they won't feed you, but they'll work hard to make you well again. They're not much help in the short run but crucial in the long run.

Sure, some medicines work over longer time frames, and some foods can have immediate optimum effects. Mostly, though, our pills and foods play different roles with respect to our health. They can be beneficial if used together, but expecting our foods to replace medication is unwise.

Superfoods can do a lot less in a month than expected and far more in a year than you may imagine. This book will show you what you can expect from super-nutrients when it comes to dealing with your lifestyle diseases and other health issues.

DIFFERENT STROKES FOR DIFFERENT FOLKS

'When the student is ready, the teacher appears,' is how the saying goes. This book meets you where you are in your journey of understanding your health. Some of the things you will find in it:

- Simple advice like how many moringa leaves to consume daily or how to select and store green tea
- A closer look at the nutrients in tomatoes or why jamuns can help in managing diabetes
- A deeper dive into the scientific world, exploring how papaya aids in combatting dengue and malaria, or why nursing mothers should avoid asafoetida
- A discussion on whether the saturated fats in coconut are harmful or why healing joint cartilage requires meeting one specific condition

Take in what you need now and save the rest for later.

SPREADING KNOWLEDGE

Finally, this book seeks to offer its health message not as a blinding floodlight but as the gentle flame of a candle – the less ostentatious of the two, yet the only one capable of lighting another candle. If you find this book useful, please pass it on to your family and friends, so that they, too, can benefit in the long run.

With that, I now hand you the keys found lying in a dim corner of the world of nutritional science. I hope they lead you to unlock the door to a healthier, more vibrant life.

1

TOMATO

Antioxidant Elixir

Is tomato a fruit or a vegetable? The United States Supreme Court disagrees with an average botany teacher's claim that tomato is a fruit.

In 1883, US President Chester A. Arthur signed a Tariff Act imposing duties on all imported vegetables, excluding fruits. This had grave consequences, as not only tomatoes but also cucumbers, pumpkins, eggplants, avocados and green beans belonged to the same category. Should they have been exempted?

New York-based importer of vegetables John Nix and Company – which imported tomatoes, among other items – refused to pay any import duty, arguing that the tomato was a fruit.

'Not possible,' responded the Port of New York Collector. With millions of dollars hanging in the balance, the court battle escalated to the Supreme Court in 1892. The judges were faced with a secondary school botany question: is the tomato a fruit or a vegetable?

There was ample confusion in the courtroom. John Nix and Company asserted that Worcester's Dictionary *defined cauliflower, potato, cabbage, carrot and beans as fruits. Given its similarity to these items, they considered the tomato a fruit. The Port of New York retorted with a citation from Webster's Dictionary, claiming eggplant, cucumber, pepper and peas to be vegetables, and argued that tomatoes were similar.*

After a year of debate and consideration, the court issued its verdict: 'Tomatoes are consumed primarily in the main course, not as a dessert. Hence, we rule that a tomato is a vegetable, and import duty must be paid on it.'

Despite this, your botany teacher will maintain that scientifically, a tomato is a fruit because it bears seeds and sprouts from a flower. Just remember the saying, 'Knowledge is knowing that a tomato is a fruit; wisdom is not putting it in your dessert.'

Tomato is the edible fleshy fruit of the nightshade plant *Solanum lycopersicum*. The name is derived from the Aztec word '*tomatl*', which gave rise to the Spanish '*tomate*'.[1] Wild varieties of tomatoes emerged in Peru and Ecuador before they were subsequently modified in Mexico a few hundred years ago and introduced to Europe by the Spanish in the sixteenth century.

Europeans once thought the tomato to be a decorative plant, believing it was poisonous and unsuitable for consumption. In those days, pewter – a tin alloy – was employed to make tableware because of its metallic lustre and the ease with which utensils could be manufactured. But the cheaper pewter vessels also contained high amounts of lead. As tomatoes are acidic, they caused lead from the pewter plates to leach into the dish. The result: numerous incidents of food poisoning.[2] Although utensils are no longer made with pewter, using aluminium containers with tomatoes warrants similar caution.

NUTRIENTS

A tomato contains 95 per cent water, 3.9 per cent carbohydrates, 0.9 per cent proteins and 0.2 per cent fats.[3]

Nutrition in Suggested Daily Amount of Tomato		Eat **100** grams
		Has **18** calories
Source	*Nutrient*	*Daily Need (%)*
Good	Vitamin C	17.5
	Vitamin K	14.4
	Vitamin B$_9$ (folate)	7.5
	Manganese	5.7
	Vitamin E	5.4
	Potassium	5.0
Poor	Vitamin A equivalent	4.2
	Vitamin B$_6$ (pyridoxine)	4.0
	Phosphorous	4.0
	Magnesium	3.7
	Vitamin B$_3$ (Niacin)	3.3
	Dietary Fibres	3.0
	Copper	3.0
	Vitamin B$_1$ (thiamine), vitamin B$_5$ (pantothenic acid), vitamin B$_2$ (riboflavin), calcium, zinc, iron, sodium and selenium	Less than 3

Unlike the claims on numerous websites, tomatoes are not a significant source of dietary fibre, providing just one gram. They are, however, abundant in healthy plant compounds known as antioxidants, which play a key role in enhancing health and longevity. Antioxidants prevent or slow the processes leading to degeneration of the body or ageing. The main antioxidant plant compounds in tomatoes include:[4]

- **Lycopene**: Contains antioxidant, anti-inflammatory, anti-cancer and anti-diabetes properties, and protects the heart, brain, bones, eyes and skin.[5] Since lycopene is found in the tomato skin, it's advisable not to peel tomatoes before eating.
- **Carotenes**: Antioxidant, anti-inflammatory, anti-cancer and anti-diabetic properties, and protects the eyes, skin, heart, brain and immune system[6]
- **Quercetin:**[7] Antioxidant,[8] anti-inflammatory,[9] anti-allergic,[10] anti-cancer[11] and brain-protective[12] properties. It is also known to guard the heart.[13]
- **Kaempferol**: Antioxidant, anti-inflammatory, anti-cancer and antimicrobial properties, with protective effects on the heart, brain, bones, liver, lungs and digestive system[14]
- **Chlorogenic acid**: Anti-inflammatory, anti-cancer, anti-diabetes and anti-obesity properties, and protects the liver and heart[15]
- **Naringin**: Found in tomato skin, and acts as an antioxidant with anti-inflammatory, anti-cancer, anti-diabetes, heart-protective and bone-protective properties[16]
- **Phytosterols:**[17] Antioxidant, anti-inflammatory,[18] anti-cancer[19] and immunity-boosting[20] properties, along with cholesterol-lowering benefits[21]

HEALTH BENEFITS

As seen above, tomatoes offer a variety of health advantages.[22] Let's delve into each of these findings.

Heart-Protective Benefits

- ✓ Diets rich in tomatoes are known to lower the risk of heart disease.[23]
- ✓ Eating tomatoes can lower the levels of cholesterol and triglycerides in our blood, while increasing HDL, also known as 'good cholesterol'.[24]
- ✓ They can reduce the quantities of blood chemicals causing inflammation and oxidative stress, which are harmful to the heart.[25]
- ✓ Tomatoes aid in lowering blood pressure.[26]
- ✓ They can bring down the blood's clotting tendencies,[27] helping prevent plaque formation in the heart arteries.[28]
- ✓ By reducing cholesterol, inflammation, blood pressure and blood-clotting tendencies, tomatoes can help ward off cardiovascular disease.[29]

Anti-Cancer Benefits

Tomatoes may provide benefits that help in preventing lung,[30] prostate[31] and breast[32] cancers. But you must carry on with your prescribed cancer treatment, even as you update your diet. Tomatoes are not a substitute for the medical management of cancer, as their benefits manifest over a longer period, making them best suited as a preventative or supportive aid.

Anti-Diabetes Benefits

- ✓ Tomatoes improve glucose and fat metabolism in diabetic patients.[33]
- ✓ They enhance the effectiveness of metformin, a common medication for diabetes.[34]
- ✓ They may aid against kidney damage, a frequent complication caused by diabetes.[35]

Eye-Protective Benefits

Consuming tomatoes is beneficial for eye health due to their eye-protective antioxidants, including lycopene, lutein, zeaxanthin and beta-carotenes. They offer the following advantages:

- ✓ They can reduce the risk of developing age-related cataracts.
- ✓ They can protect against eye damage caused by blue and ultraviolet rays.[36]
- ✓ Tomatoes can help alleviate symptoms of age-related macular degeneration (AMD), an eye disease that can blur your central vision by damaging the macula – the central part of the retina.[37]

Brain-Protective Benefits

- ✓ Tomatoes may help reduce the risk of stroke.[38]
- ✓ Lycopene has been found to be effective against various aspects of Alzheimer's disease, which affects the patient's memory.[39]
- ✓ Similarly, tomatoes and lycopene help with various problems associated with Parkinson's disease, a mobility disorder.[40]

Reproductive Benefits

- ✓ Eating tomatoes during pregnancy may prevent congenital abnormalities. Deficiency of vitamin B_9 before or during pregnancy in the mother's body can lead to birth defects. Being rich in vitamin B_9, tomatoes can counteract such deficiencies.[41] But please wash tomatoes thoroughly before consuming, as they are often sprayed with pesticides that can have toxic effects on the foetus.
- ✓ Tomatoes also enhance sperm motility,[42] which can potentially boost male fertility.

Skin-Protective Benefits

- ✓ Tomatoes, rich in vitamin C, aid in forming proteins that improve the skin's firmness and elasticity, preventing wrinkles, fine lines and sagging.[43] They thus contribute to maintaining youthful, healthy skin.[44]
- ✓ The vitamins C and E in tomatoes can also protect against skin damage caused by harmful ultraviolet rays in the sunlight.[45] Remember, applying tomatoes on your skin is not a substitute for sunscreen. Consuming them is the right way to help your skin.

Respiratory Benefits

While tomatoes don't particularly protect the lungs, they can be helpful in improving some lung conditions by reducing bodily inflammation.

- ✓ Studies indicate that tomatoes may be beneficial for people with asthma.[46]

- ✓ They may also help ward off emphysema, a condition which causes shortness of breath.[47]

Note that while this research is promising, it is still in its early stages.

Immunity Benefits

- ✓ Tomatoes bolster immunity[48], thanks to their lycopene, beta-carotene and vitamin C contents.
- ✓ They aid in fighting against external bacteria and viruses.[49]
- ✓ Tomatoes are being studied as a new type of 'edible' vaccine.[50] While this benefit is not applicable yet, it shows that tomatoes can potentially improve our immunity against many infectious diseases.

Post-Exercise Recovery Benefits

Exercise is good for general health, but it also increases energy production, leading to excess inflammation and potential damage to body proteins. Tomatoes have been found to reduce inflammation after exercise, improving recovery.[51] Recent research indicates, though, that exercise-induced inflammation actually triggers the body to rebuild and strengthen itself.

> *'What doesn't kill you makes you stronger'*
> – FRIEDRICH NIETZSCHE, nineteenth-century German philosopher

This suggests that eating tomatoes to reduce inflammation can slow down the process of exercise-induced improvements.[52] Consuming tomatoes can be beneficial for non-competitive athletes, as they can recover quicker and return to work. Professional athletes, on the other hand, should be careful since it may delay their adaptation to a greater exercise load.

Digestive Benefits

Tomatoes contain only 1.2 per cent dietary fibre by weight, making them a poor source of fibre and ineffective in alleviating constipation and other digestive system problems.

Some websites and research papers claim that as much as 11 per cent of a tomato's weight comprises dietary fibre, suggesting it is a terrific digestive aid.[53] However, since tomatoes are 95 per cent water, this can only happen with dried tomatoes.

In the suggested daily amount (**100 g**), tomatoes can't provide enough fibres to make a difference for people who are prone to constipation.

HOW TO CONSUME

Tomatoes can be eaten raw, dried, pickled or juiced. They can be cooked to create sauces, pastes, purées, ketchup or soups, and can be added to salads, salsas and dips. They can also be stuffed, baked or roasted.[54]

Generally, they pair well with beans, chillies, shrimp and cheese, and can be topped with basil, cilantro, oregano and garlic.

HOW TO SELECT

- ✓ Pick ones with firm, unwrinkled and deep red skin, without any yellow or green patches.
- ✓ A good tomato should feel heavy for its size.
- ✓ Reject any that are overly soft or leaking liquid.
- ✓ A ripe tomato should have an aromatic smell. If it has spoiled, it may develop mould. To prevent a runny or blocked nose, skin and eye irritation or wheezing, do not try to smell a visibly mouldy tomato.

HOW TO STORE

- ✓ Unripe tomatoes can be stored at room temperature, with the stem side facing down and away from direct sunlight.
- ✓ Once ripe, they will last for up to five days at room temperature.
- ✓ Tomatoes can be stored in the refrigerator for two weeks.
- ✓ Inside the deep freezer, they can last a few more months.

SHOULD YOU COOK TOMATOES?

Does cooking tomatoes make them more nutritious than eating them raw? The answer: yes and no.[55] Some nutrients are destroyed in the process of cooking. For instance, vitamin C oxidizes into biologically inactive compounds when heated. If you cook tomatoes for 15 to 30 minutes, their vitamin C content drops by 15 to 30 per cent.

On the other hand, lycopene, the most crucial antioxidant in tomatoes, is locked within the fibrous walls of its cells. On cooking, these walls break down, releasing lycopene and thus increasing the overall antioxidant levels by 30 to 60 per cent in a cooked tomato.[56] Therefore, pastes, purées and ketchup – all cooked products – are far more nutritious than raw tomatoes.

Avoid cooking tomatoes in aluminium utensils, as mentioned earlier. Also, if a cast iron vessel is not seasoned, the acid from tomatoes may interact with the iron and make the food taste metallic. Go for stainless steel vessels, as they don't react with acidic ingredients.

HOW MUCH TO CONSUME

- ✓ There is no pre-determined daily amount for it. But you can eat up to **one** medium-sized or **six** small cherry tomatoes (equivalent to **100 g**) in a day.
- ✓ It's best not to eat tomatoes every day; two to three times per week is sufficient.
- ✓ Since lycopene is a potent antioxidant, a few people eat tomatoes mainly for this particular benefit. Experts suggest consuming between **10** and **20 mg** of lycopene in a day.[57] A hundred grams of tomatoes will yield 3 mg of lycopene when uncooked and 12 mg when cooked. But do not start slurping tomato purée. While it adds to your lycopene intake, you might seem socially peculiar!
- ✓ Other sources of lycopene include watermelon, red bell peppers and papaya. This means, you don't really need to consume tomatoes every day to fulfil your lycopene needs.

HOW MUCH IS TOO MUCH

- ✓ There is no known toxic dose for tomatoes.
- ✓ One should not exceed **two** medium-sized (around **200 g**) tomatoes per day, as having too many can lead to side

effects like acidity or heartburn, bloating, diarrhoea, skin discolouration and even kidney stones.
- ✓ Experts advise against consuming more than **75 mg** of lycopene a day, an amount found in 2.5 kg of uncooked and 625 g of cooked tomatoes.

WHO SHOULD AVOID

- ✓ People with gastroesophageal reflux disease (GERD) should limit their tomato consumption due to its high malic and citric acid contents. Tomatoes can trigger excess acid secretion in the stomach, leading to heartburn and reflux.
- ✓ Anyone who is allergic to tomatoes may develop skin rashes, eczema, coughing, itchy throat, sneezing and swelling of the face and mouth on consuming them.[58] But as someone who is reading this book, you're likely old enough to know if you have a tomato allergy!
- ✓ Tomato skins and seeds can trigger bloating in patients with irritable bowel syndrome (IBS), an intestinal disorder causing diarrhoea, constipation, bloating and abdominal pain.
- ✓ Tomatoes contain some food allergens that can cause digestive issues.[59]
- ✓ Pregnant women should avoid excess tomato consumption, as it may cause pre-term labour and low-birth-weight babies.[60]
- ✓ Breastfeeding women should also restrict consumption as lycopene can be passed on to the infant through breast milk.
- ✓ We do not know the safe amount of lycopene that can be

consumed by children, so it is best not to give them too many tomatoes to eat.
- ✓ If you're taking blood-thinning medicines, don't eat too many tomatoes, as lycopene can reduce the blood's clotting tendency.
- ✓ If you are undergoing elective surgery, avoid excess tomato consumption two weeks before and after the surgery to prevent the risk of excess bleeding.
- ✓ Tomatoes may trigger headaches in people who experience migraines.[61]
- ✓ Eating too many tomatoes can give yellow-orange colouration to your skin.[62] Once you reduce the intake, though, the skin will revert to its normal pigmentation.[63]
- ✓ Since tomatoes are acidic, they may irritate the bladder, leading to urinary incontinence.[64] They can also cause a burning sensation in the bladder (cystitis).[65]
- ✓ Tomatoes can help lower blood pressure.[66] But don't overconsume them, as blood pressure-lowering medication may interact with them and reduce it more than necessary, potentially causing a fainting episode.
- ✓ They contain potassium, which also helps in controlling blood pressure. However, people with advanced kidney disease must restrict their potassium intake.
- ✓ Tomatoes are high in oxalates, naturally occurring molecules found in abundance in plants and humans. When oxalates bind to calcium during urine production, kidney stones are formed. So, eating a lot of tomatoes may even lead to kidney stones.[67]
- ✓ They also contain a compound called solanine, which is known to cause calcium accumulation in the tissues, leading to inflammation and joint pain. But unfortunately,

there is no study on tomatoes that has definitively confirmed or denied this possibility. When in doubt, stay out: if you suffer from joint pain, restrict your tomato intake.
- ✓ Tomatoes are prone to developing mould, which can lead to respiratory problems.[68]
- ✓ Commercially available tomato sauce, ketchup and tomato soup contain high amounts of sodium that is problematic for patients with high blood pressure. Look for low-sodium varieties or prepare them at home.
- ✓ Additionally, commercially available ketchup may also be very high in sugar. So, diabetics should be careful about consuming it or look for a low-sugar variety.
- ✓ Tomatoes can have a high level of pesticide residue. Therefore, either wash your tomatoes thoroughly or opt for organically grown ones.

While this is a laundry list of issues associated with tomato consumption, one need not become paranoid. Most of us will never face these problems. But it is wise to be aware of them.

SUMMARY

Systems and Benefits	Major	Minor
Anti-inflammatory	■	
Antioxidant	■	
Bones		■
Brain		■
Cancer		■
Diabetes		■
Digestive		
Eyes		■
Heart	■	
Immunity		■
Joints		■
Liver		
Mental Health		
Pregnancy & Lactation		■
Respiratory		■
Skin & Hair		■

Consumption: **One** medium-sized tomato (**100 g**) per day, two to three times weekly.

Excess: Avoid consuming more than **two** medium-sized tomatoes (**200 g**) daily.

2

GARLIC

Heart Guardian

According to Hindu mythology, Sage Durvasa once cursed the gods, robbing them of their strength. In response, the asuras, known as the anti-gods, seized the opportunity and waged war against the weakened gods, emerging victorious. Facing dire circumstances, the gods realized their sole hope for rejuvenation was amrit, the nectar of immortality, lying at the bottom of the ocean. However, retrieving this elixir would be impossible without the asuras' aid. Thus, the gods proposed to share the amrit with the asuras in exchange for their help in causing the samudra manthan *– the churning of the cosmic sea.*

Years of agitation brought forth fourteen different ratnas – gems – from the ocean, one after another. The first gem churned from the sea was halahal, *a deadly poison, and the last the much sought-after amrit. It was agreed that the gods would partake of the amrit first, and then it would be the asuras' turn. But the gods secretly plotted not to share the nectar with the asuras at all. Sensing this deceit, an asura named Svarbhanu disguised himself as a god and drank the elixir out of turn.*

At that very moment, the gods sensed the trickery and realized that Svarbhanu would become immortal if he ingested the nectar. To prevent this, they decapitated him before it could pass down his throat. As drops of amrit fell upon the earth from his mouth, garlic sprouted at that exact spot.

Even today, garlic is not used in any religious food offerings in India, in spite of its flavour and thousand-year history of therapeutic uses, as it is believed to have originated from the mouth of an asura.

As an allegory,[1] the samudra manthan represents the process of introspection that we must undertake to explore the depths of our minds, considering both our virtuous and darker aspects.

Initially, the process will yield toxic thoughts, like the halahal poison. But the ultimate result will be the elixir of blissfulness – amrit. Interestingly, the penultimate ratna to arise from the ocean was Dhanwantari, the divine physician!

The final two gems from the churn represent the most difficult achievements: health and nirvana. A landmark in Indian philosophy, the samudra manthan holds significance in terms of health and, of course, in the lore of garlic.

Garlic (scientific name *Allium sativum*), a close cousin of onions and leeks, belongs to the lily family. It has been used for centuries in various cultures as a food-flavouring agent. Moreover, it is a part of ancient, traditional and modern medicinal practices, valued for its potential to prevent and manage many health disorders.

NUTRIENTS

Fresh garlic contains 59 per cent water, 33 per cent carbohydrates, 6.3 per cent proteins and 0.5 per cent fats.[2]

Nutrition in Suggested Daily Amount of Fresh garlic		Eat **4** grams
		Has **6** calories
Source	Nutrient	Daily Need (%)
	Manganese	3.3
Poor	Vitamin B_6 (pyridoxine), vitamin C, selenium, phosphorous, calcium, copper, vitamin B_1 (thiamine), vitamin B_5 (pantothenic Acid), potassium, magnesium, vitamin B_2 (riboflavin), zinc, iron, dietary fibres, vitamin B_3 (niacin), vitamin K, vitamin B_9 (folate), sodium, vitamin E and vitamin A equivalent*	Less than 3

* This nutrient list is in decreasing percentages of their respective daily requirements.

Several websites contend that garlic is rich in vitamins B_6 and C, as well as minerals like manganese, selenium and phosphorous. Such claims are based on the nutrient table, which, as per the industry norm, details nutrient content per hundred grams of a food item. Since we cannot – and should not – eat more than a few grams of garlic daily, it is impractical to obtain enough vitamins and minerals from it.

The key benefits and distinctive aroma of garlic result from its numerous sulphur-containing compounds (organosulphurs).[3] Other beneficial contents include saponins, polysaccharides and phenolic compounds.[4]

HEALTH BENEFITS

Garlic boasts many health benefits, including serving as an antioxidant, anti-inflammatory agent and providing heart-protective, anti-cancer and antimicrobial properties.

Antioxidant Benefits

- It neutralizes damaging molecules known as free radicals that can lead to multiple degenerative diseases.[5]
- Garlic plays a role in restoring the activities of certain chemicals that guard against heart blockages, high blood pressure and brain disorders, which are often impeded by free radicals.[6]

Anti-inflammatory Benefits

It stops various inflammatory reactions that can build up in the body. By lowering inflammation, the risk of many degenerative disorders is also reduced.

Heart-Protective Benefits

Garlic is considered a superfood for heart health. Here are some ways in which it helps:

1. Lowering Cholesterol

- Reduces the the 'bad' types of cholesterol – total and LDL.[7] This is partially because garlic prevents the production of certain chemicals required to make cholesterol in our bodies.[8]
- Elevates HDL – the 'good' cholesterol.

2. Preventing Plaque Formation

- Disrupts the unhealthy oxidation of cholesterol and its tendency to stick to arterial walls.[9] Unchecked, it can combine with certain fats and calcium to form waxy deposits known as plaques in the blood arteries.[10]
- In individuals who smoke or have high blood pressure, misbehaviour of certain cells in the arterial walls causes abnormal growth, triggering plaque formation and its eventual rupture. Garlic inhibits the growth of these cells.[11]

3. Lowering Blood Pressure

- Garlic relaxes the walls of blood vessels, leading to a drop in blood pressure.[12]

Are Your Blood Vessels More Like a Rubber Hose or a Metal Pipe?

If you pump water at high pressure through a soft rubber hose, the force causes the hose to bulge slightly, relieving some of the internal pressure. But under similar

> conditions, a metal hosepipe stays rigid, not allowing any change in water pressure.
>
> The same principle applies to your blood vessels. In our younger years, arteries are more flexible. When blood pressure rises for any reason, the arteries expand just a bit, lowering the pressure. But with age or as a result of certain heart conditions, arteries may harden due to calcium and other deposits. Also, the levels of some chemicals, called vasodilators, which prevent the blood vessels from constricting, may drop. This leads to high blood pressure, as the increased pressure cannot be released by expanding arteries.

There are two natural ways to keep the blood pressure in check:
- Preserve the levels of vasodilators in artery walls
- Prevent your arteries from hardening due to deposits

Garlic aids in both these respects.

4. Reducing Blood-Clotting

When you get a cut, blood cells called platelets come together and stick to one another at the wound site. This forms a clot, which helps in healing the wound. But sometimes, even without an actual wound, platelets may form unwanted clumps in the arteries, setting off a heart attack or a stroke. Garlic reduces the tendency of platelets to cling together, lowering the risk of undesirable clot formation.[13]

Garlic safeguards heart health when consumed regularly over a long period. Eating garlic for just a few weeks may not yield the same benefits. But it is never too late to start, in order to maintain your cardiovascular system health.

Cancer-Protective Benefits

- ✓ Certain harmless chemicals become toxic once they enter our bodies. Garlic prevents them from turning cancerous.[14]
- ✓ Our liver converts toxic substances into less harmful chemicals that are easier to excrete through urine and other means. Garlic aids in detoxifying the liver and eliminating cancer-causing toxins from the body.[15]
- ✓ It prevents cancerous cells from multiplying unchecked.[16]
- ✓ Our bodies have a system to destroy cancerous cells, but some harmful cancer cells can dodge this process. Garlic can help the body in killing such evasive cells.[17]
- ✓ Once cancer tumours become larger than a few millimetres, their growth needs more nutrients. The tumour cells then start to stimulate the formation of new blood vessels. Garlic can suppress the substances required for such blood vessel generation (neoangiogenesis).[18]
- ✓ Eating more than 10 g of garlic every day may reduce the risk of prostate, colon and stomach cancers.[19] But this much garlic may also cause heartburn and other side effects, so it should be taken only under medical supervision.

Please remember not to stop your cancer treatment. While the research on garlic in relation to some cancers is promising, it's still at an early stage. You can include garlic in your diet to obtain its general health advantages, along with some possible benefits for cancers.

Immunity-Protective Benefits

✓ Garlic can reduce bacterial activity in the body.
✓ It acts as an antiviral, alleviating symptoms of cold and flu.[20]

Remember not to rely solely on garlic for treating bacterial or viral infections.

Liver-Protective Benefits

✓ It helps reduce fatty liver conditions.[21]
✓ Garlic can prevent or treat liver injury caused by chemicals such as alcohol, pollutants and toxic medicines.[22] If uncontrolled, the resulting scarring can progress to fatty liver, hepatitis, fibrosis, cirrhosis, liver failure and liver cancer.
✓ It protects your liver from damage by preserving healthy intestinal microorganisms known as gut microbiota.[23] Since many processes in our body are interlinked, improper lifestyle choices can often compromise the intestinal bacterial mass,[24] leading to harmful substances reaching the liver and thereby triggering oxidative stress and inflammation. Who would have thought that excessive stress could cause liver inflammation by altering gut microbiota? Therefore, consume garlic also for the sake of your intestinal bacteria!

Digestive Benefits

- ✓ Garlic can ease the symptoms of digestive disorders, like inflammatory bowel disease, by reducing oxidative stress and inhibiting inflammation.[25]
- ✓ It can control gastric ulcers by killing the bacteria that cause them (*H. pylori*).[26]

Anti-Diabetes Benefits[27]

- ✓ Garlic reduces average blood glucose levels or glycated haemoglobin (HbA$_1$c) in patients suffering from type 2 diabetes.[28]
- ✓ It guards against diabetic retinopathy – a long-term side effect of diabetes on vision.[29]
- ✓ It protects against diabetes by reducing oxidative stress in the pancreas and liver.[30]

Joint-Protective Benefits

Inflammation is a major cause of osteoarthritis, which causes joint pain.
- ✓ Garlic, with its anti-inflammatory properties, can prevent the development of osteoarthritis.[31]
- ✓ For centuries, garlic has been used to treat osteoarthritis.

Bone-Protective Benefits

- ✓ It reduces the levels of certain inflammation-causing chemicals in the body, preventing bone-mass breakdown.
- ✓ Garlic helps maintain bone mass after menopause.[32]

Brain-Protective Benefits

- ✓ Garlic reduces the formation of certain proteins which, when deposited in the brain, lead to Alzheimer's disease, a condition causing memory loss.[33]
- ✓ It has been seen to improve thinking and learning functions in laboratory animals being treated for Alzheimer's.[34]
- ✓ It benefits the hippocampus, a region of the brain that is responsible for learning, memory and spatial navigation.[35]

These benefits are attributed to the organo-sulphur compounds in garlic. Although these findings are exciting, they are preliminary.

Physical Performance Benefits

- ✓ Interestingly, garlic was the world's first performance-enhancing substance! Between 776 BCE and 393 CE, during the ancient Olympics, athletes were given garlic to boost their performance.
- ✓ It may improve physical performance in individuals suffering from heart damage.[36]
- ✓ Because garlic has not been shown to benefit the physical performance of modern-day elite athletes,[37] it is not featured on the list of banned substances in international sports. Well, here comes your chance of winning an Olympic medal by consuming garlic!

> **Does Garlic Drive Away Vampires?**
>
> Balkan mythology suggests that garlic can ward off vampires. To test this belief, some scientists conducted an intriguing experiment.[38]
>
> Unable to source actual blood-sucking vampires for their study, the researchers settled on the next best candidate: leeches, which are parasites known for attaching to hosts, puncturing their skin and sucking blood.[39] The scientists discovered that leeches actually preferred to latch on to a hand smeared with garlic three times quicker than to a clean hand. This led them to conclude, tongue-in-cheek, that garlic attracts vampires rather than repelling them!

HOW TO CONSUME

Garlic can be eaten raw, roasted, baked, sautéed or cooked in various dishes, whether whole, crushed or chopped. Roasting garlic enhances its flavour and sweetness, while crushing it results in a savoury and slightly bitter taste. It is used extensively in sauces, dressings, marinades, pickles and chutneys due to its versatile nature. Garlic is a staple in most Indian dishes and is featured in numerous foreign cuisines.[40] It can be paired with acidic vegetables such as tomatoes and citrus fruits, as well as poultry and seafood. Additionally, garlic complements seasonings like oregano, basil and thyme and can be consumed in many forms: fresh, aged and as a dehydrated powder or infused oil.

Fresh Garlic

Fresh, uncut garlic contains an enzyme known as alliin (yes, with two Is). Intriguingly, alliin doesn't offer any health benefits on its own. It's only when garlic is cut or chopped that alliin slowly transforms into allicin, a chemical that imbues several advantageous properties and the distinctive smell of garlic.[41]

Alliin can be deactivated easily by heating, microwaving or mixing with stomach acid, which occurs when you swallow an uncut clove. Contrarily, allicin remains stable under these conditions.

Hence, the recommended practice is to allow time for alliin to convert into allicin before using garlic. Whether you cut, chop or mince, let it sit for five to ten minutes. Once allicin has formed, garlic can be consumed as preferred: after heating, cooking or swallowing raw.

Dried Garlic Powder

For those hoping to avoid garlic breath and body odour after eating fresh garlic, dried powder or garlic tablets can serve as suitable substitutes. Given that fresh garlic is roughly 60 per cent water, the resulting powder is 40 per cent of the weight of fresh garlic.

To make dried garlic powder, fresh garlic is dehydrated and then pulverized. As the conversion of alliin to allicin requires water, this powder contains alliin. Swallowing dried garlic powder leads to the same issue as eating uncut ones: There will be no allicin production before the stomach acid destroys alliin.

When using garlic powder in cooking, avoid sprinkling it directly onto hot food, as this will inactivate alliin. Instead, mix the powder with water and allow the paste to sit for a few minutes before incorporating into your dish.

Enterically Coated Garlic Powder Tablets

To prevent stomach acid from deactivating alliin, dried garlic powder tablets are covered with a food-grade enteric coating that does not dissolve in the stomach acid, keeping the alliin intact. Later, as the tablet reaches the slightly alkaline environment of the intestines, the coating dissolves and the dried garlic powder mixes with water in the gut to form the beneficial entity – allicin.

Garlic Oil

Garlic oil, a rising favourite, is made by steam-distilling crushed garlic cloves to extract an oily distillate. This is then blended with vegetable oils, yielding a commercially accessible preparation.

If you make garlic oil at home, you must store it carefully. If left unrefrigerated, it can turn poisonous due to the growth of lethal botulism bacteria.[42]

Spores of anaerobic bacteria called *Clostridium botulinum* can sometimes adhere to minuscule soil particles on garlic, even after a thorough wash. These spores can't thrive in the presence of oxygen. But when garlic is covered with oil, the oxygen-free environment triggers the bacteria to produce the poisonous botulinum toxin. Without prompt treatment, one-third of botulism patients die.

Aged-Garlic Extract

The healthiest, albeit the most cumbersome option, is aged-garlic extract. To prepare it, garlic is immersed in water with 20 per cent alcohol and kept at low temperatures for twenty months. This process eliminates the pungent garlic smell by converting most of its smelly substances into other beneficial but non-odorous chemicals. Moreover, aged garlic contains some new compounds that exhibit far better antioxidant capabilities than those in fresh garlic.[43]

HOW TO SELECT[44]

- ✓ Squeeze the garlic heads. Fresh bulbs will feel firm, while older heads may be soft or dry.
- ✓ Yellowed cloves are usable, though their best days may be behind them.
- ✓ Avoid sprouting bulbs (those with bright green shoots coming out the top of cloves). While edible, they have a bitter taste. If you have already bought them, cut off the shoots before use.

HOW TO STORE[45]

- ✓ Keep full garlic bulbs in a ventilated, cool and dry place (approximately 18°C [65°F]) so that they can last up to six months.
- ✓ Store in an open basket to allow dry air circulation. Avoid using plastic bags, which can seal the moisture inside. Humidity is garlic's nemesis, as it can lead to sprouting and rot by way of mould. Full garlic bulbs should never be stored inside the refrigerator.

- ✓ Smaller garlic heads have a longer storage life.
- ✓ Do not separate the cloves if you want to store garlic for a long time. Once the cloves are detached, if their papery peel is intact, they should be used within three weeks.
- ✓ Peeled garlic cloves, though, need to be stored inside the refrigerator and can be used for up to a week. Store them inside a sealed bag or plastic container to retain moisture.
- ✓ Chopped, minced or cut cloves of garlic should be only kept for a day inside the refrigerator.[46] You should smear oil over them to extend their life by an additional day or two. Any longer, and the oil can develop mould.
- ✓ Commercially available garlic pastes contain preservatives, which can extend their shelf life. Always check the expiry date and storage instructions printed on the packaging.

HOW MUCH TO CONSUME

There is no specific daily requirement for garlic; however, here are the suggested dosages:[47]

Form	Daily Dose (mg)
Fresh raw garlic	2,000–5,000
Dried garlic powder	400–1,200
Garlic oil concentrate	2–5
Garlic extract (solid)	300–1,000
Aged-garlic extract (liquid)	2,400–7,200

A typical garlic bulb has ten to twelve cloves. Each clove weighs 2 to 4 g, though some may be as heavy as 7 g.

As a rule of thumb, consume either **4 g** (**two** cloves) of fresh garlic, or **1 g** of dried garlic powder or **7 g** of aged-garlic extract daily. The dried powder is best consumed as **300 mg** of enterically coated tablets thrice a day.[48]

HOW MUCH IS TOO MUCH

- ✓ Consuming excessive amounts of raw garlic on an empty stomach can cause acidity, stomach upset and gas trouble. It may even harm the healthy population of intestinal bacteria.
- ✓ Avoid consuming more than **6 g** of fresh garlic in a day.
- ✓ Exceeding 15 g of fresh garlic per day can lead to toxicity, potentially resulting in internal bleeding or other side effects.
- ✓ Aged garlic, being less pungent than raw garlic, is generally gentler on the digestive system. However, it is best not to consume more than **20 g** of it in a day.

WHO SHOULD AVOID

- ✓ Those who work in people-facing industries, such as hospitality and sales, due to common side effects like garlic breath and body odour.
- ✓ Anyone allergic to garlic[49]
- ✓ Anyone on anti-clotting medicines, reducing the risk of unwanted bleeding[50]
- ✓ Anyone undergoing elective surgery should avoid garlic two weeks before and after the surgery to minimize the risk of excessive bleeding.
- ✓ The effects of garlic consumption during pregnancy or while breastfeeding are not well understood. Therefore, it's better not to exceed **2 g** of garlic in a day to remain on the safe side.

SUMMARY

Systems and Benefits	Major	Minor
Anti-inflammatory	■	
Antioxidant	■	
Bones		■
Brain		■
Cancer	■	
Diabetes		■
Digestive		■
Eyes		
Heart	■	
Immunity	■	
Joints		■
Liver		■
Mental Health		
Pregnancy & Lactation		
Reproductive		
Respiratory		
Skin & Hair		

Consumption: **4 g** of fresh garlic, **1 g** of dried powder, or **7 g** of aged garlic a day.

Excess: Don't consume more than **6 g** a day.

3

CINNAMON
Diabetes Warrior

Nearly three thousand years ago, cinnamon was a coveted condiment, renowned for its exotic flavour and fragrance. Royal families across Europe sought cinnamon, both for gifting and as offerings to the gods.

The cinnamon trade passed through the ancient city of Byzantium, later known as Constantinople and now Istanbul. From there, Venetian traders brought cinnamon into Europe via the Nile River and the Red Sea. However, only a small coterie of brokers knew that cinnamon originated in the jungles of Indonesia and Ceylon, which is present-day Sri Lanka. Constantinople guarded the secret of the cinnamon trade for over 2,000 years.

In 1453 CE, Constantinople fell to Ottoman forces, forcing Europeans to relinquish control over the cinnamon trade. Soon, the Asian origin of cinnamon became widely known.

The business was so lucrative that the colonial powers of Europe began looking for an alternative way to reach Asia. The king of Portugal tasked his sea explorers with finding a passage around Africa. Many attempts failed until one man triumphed:

Vasco da Gama. On 14 June 1498, the Portuguese ships sailed into the Indian port of Calicut after circumnavigating the African continent.

Subsequently, Dutch, Danish, British, French and Spanish ships followed the same route. Eventually, British forces gained control over the Indian subcontinent.

The revelation of the cinnamon trade's secret triggered the imperial powers to explore alternate routes to Asia, paving way for the British colonization of India. Thus, cinnamon played a part in shaping India's modern history.

Cinnamon (scientific name *Cinnamomum zeylanicum*) is a spice that has been widely used for thousands of years. It is a popular addition to various cuisines for its distinctive flavour and aroma. Many cultures around the world incorporate cinnamon into both sweet and savoury dishes. Not only is it known for its culinary use, it also boasts certain beneficial compounds that infuse it with medicinal properties.

NUTRIENTS

Cinnamon powder contains 11 per cent water, 81 per cent carbohydrates, 4 per cent proteins and 1.2 per cent fats.[1]

Nutrition in Suggested Daily Amount of **Cinnamon**		Eat **4** grams
		Has **10** calories
Source	*Nutrient*	*Daily Need (%)*
Great	*Manganese*	35.0
Good	*Dietary Fibres*	5.3
	Calcium	4.0
Poor	*Vitamin K, iron, vitamin E, magnesium, copper, phosphorous, zinc, potassium, vitamin B_6 (pyridoxine), selenium, vitamin B_3 (Niacin), vitamin C, vitamin B_9 (folate), vitamin B_2 (riboflavin), vitamin A equivalent, vitamin B_1 (thiamine), sodium and vitamin B_5 (pantothenic acid)*	Less than 3

Some websites claim that cinnamon is loaded with vitamins K, E and B_6, and minerals like calcium, iron, zinc and magnesium. But these claims, based on a daily serving of 100 g, misrepresent reality. Most people consume a few grams of cinnamon per day, which makes it an inadequate source of vitamins and minerals, except for manganese.

Nearly half of cinnamon is comprised of dietary fibre, providing around 2 g of fibre a day. This might make you wonder how cinnamon powder simultaneously contains 81 per cent carbohydrates and 53 per cent fibres. This is because dietary fibres are also considered carbohydrates. They are non-digestible carbohydrates (NCD), meaning our bodies cannot break them down.[2]

But certain water-soluble fibres are fermented and processed by the good bacteria in our colon. They subsequently produce, through their metabolic waste, beneficial fats known as short-chain fatty acids (SCFAs), which are absorbed in our intestines.[3] So, even though we can't digest these fibres, we derive some calories from them.

Cinnamon contains some plant compounds with significant health properties:

- ✓ **Cinnamaldehyde:** The main active ingredient found in cinnamon bark, cinnamaldehyde has anti-inflammatory, anti-bacterial and blood-pressure-lowering properties.[4] It is the source of both the pungent taste and scent of cinnamon, as well as its medicinal benefits.
- ✓ **Eugenol:** Found in the leaves and bark of the cinnamon tree, eugenol contains antioxidant, anti-inflammatory, anti-cancer, antimicrobial and pain-relieving properties.[5]

HEALTH BENEFITS

Thanks to its antioxidant and anti-inflammatory compounds, cinnamon can help manage diabetes, heart disease, cancer, certain infections and some neurodegenerative diseases.[6]

Antioxidant Benefits

- ✓ Cinnamon exhibits various antioxidant effects in the human body.[7]
- ✓ Regular use of cinnamon in food can help prevent or control many degenerative illnesses, including heart disease, diabetes, cancer and memory loss.
- ✓ Out of twenty-six different common spices, cinnamon contains the highest amount of antioxidants.[8]

Anti-inflammatory Benefits

Dozens of studies have shown that cinnamon possesses anti-inflammatory properties.[9]

Inflammation is equivalent to a hostile environment, which can be caused in many ways. While your body's immune system creates inflammation to destroy pathogens – similar to fumigating the house for pest control – energy production in body cells also causes unwanted inflammation, like your oven heating the whole kitchen.

Various anti-inflammatory compounds maintain a check on these processes. But no single nutrient can block all inflammation-causing mechanisms. This is why it is a good idea to consume several anti-inflammatory foods. This book, for instance, also examines the anti-inflammatory properties of garlic, ginger, turmeric and green tea, besides cinnamon.

It is critical to understand that not all inflammatory actions in the body should be stopped. Natural inflammatory processes help in healing wounds and controlling infections. The goal should be to prevent only excess and prolonged inflammation.

Diabetes-Protective Benefits

Cinnamon helps in blood glucose control through five different mechanisms:
- ✓ **Slowing down carbohydrate digestion:** Cinnamon inhibits the actions of enzymes involved in digesting carbohydrates,[10] effectively minimizing the glucose produced during digestion.

- ✓ **Slowing down stomach emptying:** Research indicates that cinnamon can also reduce the speed at which the stomach empties down, in turn lowering blood glucose levels after meals.[11] Normally, it takes two hours for food to transition from the stomach to the small intestine – known as the gastric emptying rate (GER). If the stomach empties too quickly, it can lead to a rapid increase in the post-meal blood glucose level.[12] Slowing down this process is beneficial for controlling blood glucose,[13] and cinnamon can achieve this without compromising satiety.
- ✓ **Lowering insulin resistance:** Cinnamon is known to lower insulin resistance, the primary cause of type 2 diabetes.[14] When body cells become less responsive to insulin, they can't fully utilize glucose for energy, pushing up blood glucose levels. This condition progressively worsens until the insulin-producing cells in the pancreas are depleted or dead. Lowering insulin resistance is vital in preventing or managing diabetes. This benefit is likely due to cinnamon's chromium content and helpful compounds called polyphenols.[15]
- ✓ **Mimicking insulin action:** Some compounds in cinnamon can act like insulin. They help our body cells use blood glucose effectively, thus lowering its levels.[16] Cinnamon can also improve the utilization of insulin.[17] Because diabetes is characterized by inadequate insulin, and the existing insulin is ineffective due to resistance, this is a valuable benefit for diabetics.
- ✓ **Controlling blood sugar:** Studies show that cinnamon can lower blood sugar levels by 10 to 30 per cent.[18] Using cinnamon has been found to achieve blood sugar reductions that align with the American Diabetes

Association's (ADA) treatment goals, which is a significant achievement.

Heart-Protective Benefits

- ✓ Cinnamon can help lower blood pressure,[19] reducing the risk of heart and vascular disorders such as strokes, eye complications, kidney damage and memory loss.
- ✓ It has been observed to lower triglycerides, total cholesterol and low-density lipoprotein (LDL) cholesterol,[20] all of which can escalate the risk of heart disease.
- ✓ High quantities of certain inflammatory chemicals in the blood suggest an increased risk of heart disease, which can be reduced by consuming cinnamon.[21]
- ✓ It can potentially protect against excessive blood clotting.[22]
- ✓ By lowering blood pressure, inflammatory chemicals, our blood's clotting tendencies, and triglyceride and cholesterol levels, cinnamon can help protect against heart disease.
- ✓ Cinnamon might also aid in reducing the harmful effects of heart attacks.[23]

Please note, it is critical to consult your doctor before starting any treatment. Also, do not try any therapy on your own against heart attacks.

Brain-Protective Benefits

- ✓ Cinnamon protects against strokes due to its compounds that have antioxidant, anti-inflammatory and blood pressure-lowering properties.

- ✓ Certain compounds in cinnamon can prevent the onset of Alzheimer's disease, which is associated with memory loss.[24]
- ✓ Moreover, its compounds can safeguard against another degenerative disorder – Parkinson's disease.[25]

Cancer-Protective Benefits

Cinnamon is being studied for its potential benefits in cancer prevention and protection.[26] While research is ongoing, there are promising findings about its capabilities.

- ✓ Cinnamon can kill abnormal cells that can become cancerous.[27] Under certain conditions where the body's immune system falls short, cinnamon could serve as a second line of defence.
- ✓ As a cancer tumour develops, its cells need additional nutrients and stimulate the region to develop new blood vessels. The compounds in cinnamon can inhibit this process, called neoangiogenesis ('neo', indicating new or additional; 'angio', meaning blood vessel; and 'genesis', implying birth) around the cancer cells.[28]
- ✓ It can prevent the unchecked growth of cancer cells.[29]
- ✓ Cancer cells can relocate from one region and grow in another body part in a process called cancer metastasis. Cinnamon can help prevent specific mechanisms involved in this process.[30]
- ✓ Some research suggests that cinnamon may be helpful when dealing with certain kinds of cancers, such as those affecting the skin,[31] colon[32] and ovaries[33].

However, cinnamon is not a primary treatment for cancer – patients should strictly follow their doctors' prescription. Discuss with them whether cinnamon can be incorporated as supportive therapy in your treatment plan. Proceed only upon their approval.

Immunity-Protective Benefits

- ✓ Cinnamon is effective against many microbial infections.[34] Although it cannot cure them, regular consumption of cinnamon can prevent frequent infections.
- ✓ It has been found helpful in treating stubborn fungal infections.[35]
- ✓ Cinnamon is also beneficial in managing various respiratory infections.[36]
- ✓ It has been found to help combat viruses causing HIV, influenza and dengue.[37]

Oral Health Benefits

- ✓ Cinnamon prevents bad breath by killing odour-causing bacteria in the mouth[38] – a key reason you will often find cinnamon-flavoured chewing gums or mouth fresheners.
- ✓ It can help ward off gum disease.
- ✓ It is effective against bacteria that cause tooth cavities. Studies have shown cinnamon exhibits better efficacy than clove oil in treating tooth decay (dental caries).[39]

Cinnamon oil is beneficial for oral health.[40] But overuse of cinnamon, particularly its oil, can cause irritation in the mouth due to its strong potency.[41]

Bone-Protective Benefits

✓ Consuming cinnamon in high quantities has been found to strengthen bones.[42]
✓ Ageing increases bone loss, leading to fragile bones. The compounds in cinnamon can help slow down this process.[43]

Both of the above benefits are due to the anti-inflammatory compounds in cinnamon. Recent scientific evidence suggests that premature bone weakness is caused by inflammation-induced bone mass breakdown rather than calcium deficiency.[44]

It is essential to note that the trials referenced above used high doses of cinnamon, which should be taken only under medical supervision. However, regular cinnamon intake may still offer some of its potential bone-protective benefits.

Liver-Protective Benefits

Cinnamon can effectively reduce the excessive enzyme levels associated with a condition known as non-alcoholic fatty liver disease (NAFLD).[45]

HOW TO CONSUME

How to Select

Four major varieties of cinnamon are commercially available in the market, each with distinct medicinal and culinary benefits:

- Ceylon Cinnamon: Grown in Sri Lanka (formerly Ceylon) and southern parts of India
- Chinese Cinnamon (Chinese Cassia)
- Indonesian Cinnamon (Padang Cassia)
- Saigon Cinnamon (Vietnamese Cassia)

Ceylon cinnamon, also known as 'true cinnamon', is considered a premium variety that is more expensive compared to the other three, which are collectively called 'cassia' due to their relatively inferior quality.[46] They are not even classified as cinnamon.

- ✓ Regulatory bodies like the Food Safety and Standards Authority of India (FSSAI) regard cinnamon and cassia as separate food items. The rules dictate that if cassia is used in a food product, it cannot be labelled as cinnamon.[47]
- ✓ Medicinally, cassia cannot match the benefits of ceylon cinnamon, but it has some useful culinary purposes. It has a high percentage of a pungent, oily compound – cinnamaldehyde – primarily responsible for cinnamon's aroma and flavour. Cassia contains around 95 per cent cinnamaldehyde, compared to ceylon cinnamon's 60 per cent.[48] Cassia tends to be strong and peppery in taste, while the other variety is sweeter.
- ✓ In everyday cooking and industrial food production, cassia is often preferred as it is nearly ten times cheaper than ceylon cinnamon. Conversely, ceylon cinnamon is reserved for desserts and for creating more delicate flavours.
- ✓ In terms of health benefits, ceylon cinnamon is considered far superior to cassia. In fact, consuming the latter in therapeutic doses can be unsafe, as will be elaborated later in this chapter.

How to Distinguish between Cassia and Ceylon Cinnamons

- ✓ Ceylon cinnamon sticks are lighter brown with thin, papery, crumply layers, while cassia cinnamon rolls are reddish and dark brown. With thick and hard-rolled bark layers, they can be easily distinguished in stick form.
- ✓ When ground to a powder, an untrained eye won't be able to tell the difference between the two.[49]
- ✓ As a general guideline, always check the product label. If it only mentions 'cinnamon' without specifying the type, it is likely cassia. A supplier using ceylon cinnamon will proudly announce it on the packaging. In India, though, the rules specify that cassia cannot be labelled as cinnamon.

HOW TO STORE

- ✓ The shelf life of cinnamon varies based on its form (powder or stick) and storage conditions.
- ✓ Cinnamon can be stored for one to two years in powdered form, and as sticks, two to four years.[50] Once ground into powder, however, it can lose its delicate oils faster as more surface area becomes exposed to air, moisture, light or heat.
- ✓ Cinnamon packets carry a 'Best Before Date' rather than an 'Expiry Date' as, although cinnamon doesn't spoil after that date, it may lose some aroma and flavour. Here's a tip: you can keep your cinnamon for up to a year beyond its 'Best Before Date' by using a larger quantity for the same aroma and flavour.

To extend the life of stored cinnamon, you can:
- ✓ Store it in a cool, dark place, as light can speed up degradation.
- ✓ Avoid storing cinnamon above your fridge or near the cooking range where it can be exposed to heat.
- ✓ Store it in a temperature-stable area. If the storage temperatures fluctuate between hot and cold, the consequent condensation can spoil the cinnamon. Don't keep your everyday-use cinnamon in the fridge for the same reason.
- ✓ Use an airtight box to protect it from moisture.
- ✓ For longer storage, use opaque glass or stainless-steel containers instead of plastic ones, as the latter can absorb odours.

Discard old cinnamon if it develops mould, moisture, wet spots or large clumps. To check, crumble some of it between your fingers and assess the aroma and flavour. If it lacks either, dispose of the cinnamon.

HOW MUCH TO CONSUME

One teaspoon of cinnamon powder roughly equals 2 g of cinnamon. Most clinical trials use between 1 and 6 g of cinnamon daily. Therefore, that is the amount to be consumed for health benefits.
- If you're using ceylon cinnamon, you can consume around **4 g (2 tsp)** in a day.[51]
- For cassia, it is recommended to stay under **0.5 g (¼ tsp)** per day, for reasons explained later in this chapter. This effectively means it is unsuitable for health and medicinal purposes.

HOW MUCH IS TOO MUCH

While both the varieties share numerous beneficial compounds, cassia contains one harmful element – coumarin – which practically rules out its medicinal use.

Coumarin

Coumarin inhibits vitamin K formation, reducing blood clotting and making it useful in some blood clot-preventing medications, such as warfarin.[52] Consuming cassia cinnamon can, therefore, increase the risk of excessive bleeding.

Moreover, high concentrations of coumarin are also known to lead to cancers and damage the liver and kidneys.[53] In severe instances, it can induce liver inflammation, resulting in jaundice symptoms.[54]

The European Food Safety Authority (EFSA) has suggested a maximum tolerable daily intake (TDI) of 100 µg of coumarin per kilogram of body weight.[55] So, a person weighing 60 kg should consume at most 6,000 µg of coumarin daily. Ceylon cinnamon contains up to 90 µg of coumarin per gram, setting the upper daily limit for consuming ceylon cinnamon at **67 g** for a sixty-kilogram person.

In contrast, cassia cinnamon contains between 2,500 and 10,000 µg of coumarin per gram,[56] nearly a hundred times more than ceylon cinnamon. This means the daily intake for cassia should be less than a gram.[57] Because of cassia's affordability and wide availability, most people unknowingly surpass the safe levels when consuming it through regular food. Hence, caution is especially advised when using it at home.

It's worth noting that research on cinnamon typically involves daily doses of 1 to 6 g. Unfortunately, many scientific papers state that the scientists conducting the study used the cassia variety. It begs the question why such researchers do not do their toxicity homework before conducting these trials!

One possible reason is that these trials are done only over a few weeks, while the risks of coumarin typically manifest after months or years of regular intake. This is also why one should not blindly adopt clinical findings and dosages without consulting an expert for advice.

WHO SHOULD AVOID

Cassia cinnamon

- ✓ People allergic to cinnamon should refrain from excessive use, as cassia is extremely potent and can cause mouth sores.[58]
- ✓ Those diagnosed with liver problems should abstain from consuming cassia, as coumarin can damage their liver further.
- ✓ People taking blood-thinning medication should avoid cassia, because coumarin may interfere with blood clotting.

Additionally, here are the precautionary measures concerning the use of all cinnamon varieties:
- ✓ People on diabetes medicines should inform their doctors if they consume cinnamon to manage their blood sugar levels. Coupled with diabetes medicines, cinnamon can lead to hypoglycaemia, a life-threatening level of low blood glucose.

- ✓ Pregnant and breastfeeding women should avoid excess cinnamon consumption.[59] While it is unclear whether cinnamon can induce pre-term labour or pose risk to a nursing infant, it's advisable to steer clear when in doubt.

SUMMARY

Systems and Benefits	Major	Minor
Anti-inflammatory	■	
Antioxidant	■	
Bones		■
Brain		■
Cancer		■
Diabetes	■	
Digestive		■
Eyes		
Heart	■	
Immunity	■	
Joints		
Liver		■
Mental Health		
Pregnancy & Lactation		
Reproductive		
Respiratory		
Skin & Hair		

Consumption: **4 g** (**2 tsp**) of ceylon cinnamon a day. Less than **1 g** of cassia a day.

Excess: Consume less than **6 g** of ceylon cinnamon or **1 g** of cassia daily.

4

GREEN TEA
Modern-Day Sanjeevani

Can a plant save you from dying? A story from the Ramayana suggests so. During a fierce battle in Lanka (today's Sri Lanka) between Ram and Ravan's forces, Ram's brother Lakshman was critically wounded and fell down unconscious. The only hope for his recovery was the magical herb – the sanjeevani – which held the power to revive the dying. But this plant existed on Mount Dronagiri in the Himalaya, thousands of kilometres away from the battlefield.

Consequently, Hanuman was dispatched to secure this herb. He began his search on Gandhamardan, a hillock near Dronagiri that was brimming with medicinal plants. Overwhelmed by the plethora of herbs there, Hanuman could not identify the correct plant. As time pressed on, he decided to carry the entire hillock to the battlefield. The subsequent application of the herb revived Lakshman from his coma, allowing him to rejoin the fight.[1]

Whether this story is a myth or reality is up for interpretation. But interestingly, a hill called the Gandhamardhan exists at present in the southeastern state of Odisha, considerably closer to the mythical battle site than the Himalaya. One can find over 500 medicinal herbs flourishing on this hill.[2]

Similarly, in the Himalayan state of Uttarakhand is Mount Dronagiri. Located twenty kilometres from it is the popular trekking destination – the Valley of Flowers, which is also famous for 500 different medicinal plants! Could it be that Hanuman brought the Gandhamardhan hill from Uttarakhand, leaving behind what we call the Valley of Flowers?

The identity of the modern sanjeevani herb remains a mystery. Despite thorough textual examination, ancient scriptures have provided no clarity, and the scientific community continues its search for answers.[3]

One senior botanist and researcher has offered a simpler proposition, claiming that the sanjeevani was in fact green tea. Considering the comparable neuro-protective properties of green tea and the mythical abilities of the sanjeevani plant in restoring dying brain nerves, he might not be wrong.

Green tea is made from the unfermented leaves of the *Camellia sinensis* plant, which also produces black tea. While its origins can be traced back to China, its popularity has since spread throughout Asia and the rest of the world. Ancient Chinese literature attests to its use for over 1,500 years.[4]

Green Tea versus Black Tea

Tea leaves are either steamed or pan-fried after harvest to produce green tea or are left to dry naturally to produce black tea. The heating process 'cooks' the leaves,[5] preventing oxidation – a reaction that blackens the leaves' green pigment.[6] Heated tea leaves retain their green colour even after they are dried, preserving the delicate natural compounds in the leaves. Voilà! You have green tea.

If the fresh tea leaves are not heated, though, they ferment and turn black. Once dried, they become black tea leaves. Many of the original compounds in the tea leaves oxidize and lose some of their health benefits during this process. They do, however, also develop a stronger aroma and tangier flavour than green tea. To draw an analogy from the world of alcohol, black tea is the country liquor to green tea's single malt.

NUTRIENTS

Brewed green tea is 99.93 per cent water,[7] which means it contains no carbohydrates, proteins or fats to write home about. But does this imply that the vitamins and minerals offered by it are insignificant, too? On the contrary, green tea is an excellent source of manganese and vitamin B_2 when used in the amounts recommended for daily consumption.

Nutrition in Suggested Daily Amount of Green tea		Drink **750** ml
		Has **7** calories
Source	*Nutrient*	*Daily Need (%)*
Great	*Manganese*	69.0
	Vitamin B_2 (riboflavin)	28.1
	Vitamin B_1 (thiamine)	3.8
Poor	*Vitamin C, magnesium, vitamin B_6 (pyridoxine), copper, potassium, vitamin B_3 (niacin), iron, sodium, zinc, dietary fibres, vitamin A equivalent, vitamin B_5 (pantothenic acid), vitamin B_9 (folate), vitamin E, vitamin K, calcium, phosphorous and selenium*	Less than 3

Green tea has many potent plant compounds. The three superstars of Team Green Tea are:

- ✓ **Catechins:** Contain antioxidant, anti-inflammatory, brain-protective, anti-bacterial, anti-viral, anti-allergenic, anti-diabetic and anti-cancer properties[8]
- ✓ **Caffeine:** Increases alertness, reduces fatigue, suppresses appetite and lowers risks of heart failure and colon cancer. It also has brain-protective,[9] anti-diabetic and liver-protective properties[10].
- ✓ **L-Theanine:** A calming agent found exclusively in green tea.[11] It helps increase feelings of happiness and motivation.[12]

HEALTH BENEFITS

Green tea's delicate catechin compounds provide numerous benefits. But not all catechins can be extracted from the leaves into the brew simultaneously during steeping. A cup of green tea contains varying amounts of catechins depending on the preparation time.

Moreover, catechins are unstable. So, simply telling people to drink green tea and then measuring the results is not a reliable way to prove its health benefits.

Brain-Protective Benefits

- ✓ Drinking green tea induces feelings of calmness, enthusiasm and happiness – subjective emotions shared by most regular green tea drinkers. This is primarily due to the presence of l-theanine, which raises the levels of

chemicals called neurotransmitters – serotonin, dopamine and GABA – in the brain.[13]
- ✓ Green tea helps lower the risk of stroke.[14]
- ✓ Its benefits may extend to individuals suffering from anxiety-related disorders – including social or generalized anxiety or obsessive-compulsive disorders (OCD) – due to l-theanine.[15]
- ✓ Green tea aids in slowing brain ageing through its catechins, which activate brain cells, and l-theanine, which can lower stress levels.[16]
- ✓ A recent study showed that catechins can also prevent brain degeneration by protecting the nerve cells in the brain.[17]

In fact, the brain-protective properties of green tea are so significant, we will first explain some essential terms related to it in more detail here.

Natural Brain Ageing[18]

- ✓ After the age of thirty years, the brain starts to shrink in size.
- ✓ With age, the production of neurotransmitters drops. Since brain nerve cells use them for communication, their interaction reduces.
- ✓ Brain nerve cells start dying with age.

Premature Brain Ageing

In some people, the brain can age faster due to oxidative stress, which leads to chronic inflammation around the brain cells (neuroinflammation), creating a fertile ground for degenerative disorders. The brain is particularly vulnerable to oxidative stress due to the following reasons:

- ✓ It accounts for 20 per cent of the body's energy needs. Since the process of energy production generates many free radicals, the brain cells face a continuous barrage of them.
- ✓ Nerve cell membranes have significant amounts of unsaturated fats vulnerable to oxidation and, therefore, damage.
- ✓ The brain lacks significant amounts of antioxidants to defend itself against neuroinflammation.

Degenerative Brain Diseases

Natural or premature brain ageing causes two main types of neurodegenerative brain disorders:

- ✓ Loss of memory (dementias, such as Alzheimer's disease)
- ✓ Loss of mobility (Parkinson's disease)

If the brain ages solely due to natural causes, both Alzheimer's and Parkinson's diseases take such a long time to develop that most people die before experiencing their symptoms. But with premature brain ageing, these two disorders can occur much earlier in life, necessitating prevention and management. One solution is to maintain high levels of antioxidants and anti-inflammatory compounds in the brain throughout the life.

But the brain is a tough nut to crack, literally.

Blood-Brain Barrier

It is not easy for most outside substances to reach the brain. With its critical role in our survival, the brain is heavily guarded and fortified. It is encased within a ten-millimetre-thick skull, surrounded by a protective fluid and three layers of protective tissues. Besides, our brain has evolved a unique mechanism – the blood-brain barrier (BBB) – to shield it from blood-borne chemicals and pathogens, allowing only a few external compounds to reach the brain cells.

Catechins are among the few antioxidants that can cross the BBB and, therefore, help suppress neurodegenerative brain diseases.[19]

Dementia

Many dementias involve memory loss and diminished cognitive skills. They can have far-reaching consequences for independent living, causing behavioural changes and interpersonal relationship issues.

Alzheimer's Disease

Alzheimer's disease accounts for 70 per cent of dementia cases. This progressive condition is marked by symptoms worsening over time. Because it first affects the brain's learning centres, early symptoms include difficulty remembering new information. As the disease progresses, symptoms grow in severity, including disorientation, confusion and behavioural changes. Eventually, even basic functions like speaking, swallowing and walking become difficult to perform.

The precise cause or triggers of Alzheimer's remain unclear, though we know it involves malfunctioning brain cells. Neuroinflammation is considered one of the miscreants.[20] We don't know whether it directly causes or worsens the problem, but it is observed to be present as the disease develops.

Many studies show the benefits of green tea on memory loss and Alzheimer's. While the exact mechanism still remains to be understood, scientists propose four possible ways green tea could help:[21]

- ✓ Antioxidant activity[22]
- ✓ Anti-inflammatory activity[23]
- ✓ Preventing the accumulation of protein waste products[24]
- ✓ Keeping the brain's blood vessels healthy[25]

Parkinson's Disease

Parkinson's disease affects the part of the brain that regulates movement and muscle control. It causes a progressive loss of mobility as well as symptoms such as tremors and jerky movement. Slower thinking and memory loss can also occur as the condition worsens.

The disease is caused by an abnormal buildup of a protein in brain nerve cells that produce dopamine – the neurotransmitter that controls our movements. The brain's immune system sees these protein deposits as threats and attacks them, releasing inflammation-causing chemicals to destroy them.

Neuroinflammation increases around those brain cells, disrupting dopamine production. As dopamine levels fall, it leads to abnormal walking, slowed movement and stiff muscles.

Furthermore, the inflammation kills some brain cells and causes oxidative stress, giving rise to more dangerous compounds. This quickly escalates neuroinflammation. The chain reaction continues, and the situation worsens. This is usually the end stage of the disease.

- ✓ Regular green tea drinkers were found to have up to 41 per cent lower incidence of Parkinson's.[26] Catechins and caffeine are believed to contribute to this effect.
- ✓ Consuming two cups of green tea every day decreases the risk of Parkinson's by 26 per cent.[27]
- ✓ Catechins reduce oxidative stress and inflammation, prevent brain cell death and improve brain cell energy production.[28] These mechanisms provide essential protection against Parkinson's disease.

Energy-Related Benefits

Green tea, like any other tea or coffee, has the ability to boost alertness. This benefit comes from its caffeine content, which is a well-known stimulant. But how exactly does it work?

How Does Caffeine Make Us Feel Fresh?

Our body's cellular metabolism produces a chemical called adenosine, which plays a role in regulating our sleep. It can attach to nerve cells in the brain, slowing their activity and making us groggy.[29]

The more active we are, the more adenosine our brain produces. So, after a number of hours of being awake, sleep is induced. Typically, sleeping is the only way to lower adenosine levels and feel rejuvenated.

Caffeine, however, has a structure that is similar to adenosine's. It attaches to brain cells at specific locations where adenosine can bind. As a result, brain cells continue to function normally. It's as if a random key is inserted into a lock, blocking the real key's entry.

As long as caffeine is locked to a brain cell, adenosine cannot attach to it, ensuring alertness. The more caffeine-attached are the cells, the fresher you feel.

But, over time, the liver keeps breaking down caffeine, lowering its concentration in our blood. Some caffeine molecules detach themselves from brain cells and return to the blood. Adenosine quickly attaches to newly freed brain cells, and you start becoming sleepy again. Since your adenosine levels would have increased in the interim, you feel drowsier than before.

The alertness induced by drinking tea or coffee is temporary and borrowed from the future. If you have a long-term deadline, avoid using caffeine to get energy. But in situations where you need to increase your attention span in the short term, like for an upcoming presentation or exam, tea or coffee might be helpful.

- ✓ Caffeine boosts memory, mood and alertness. But you don't need this book to tell you that!
- ✓ Green tea provides a gentler burst of energy than coffee. There are multiple reasons for it. Firstly, a cup of green tea has just one-third caffeine compared to a similar-sized cup of coffee. It also contains l-theanine, which not only enhances comprehension, learning skills and memory, but also reduces stress and mental fatigue, boosts feelings of calm and alertness and enhances creativity.[30] Sounds incredible? Hold on, it gets better.
- ✓ When combined with caffeine, l-theanine provides even more benefits. So you can expect improved alertness, focus, mental endurance and stress reduction from green tea compared to taking caffeine or l-theanine separately.[31]
- ✓ One drawback of caffeine is that it can raise blood pressure. However, when combined with l-theanine, this harmful effect is mitigated.[32] Unlike coffee, tea contains l-theanine, which is why it is considered a better choice than coffee for people who are under extreme stress or have high blood pressure.[33]
- ✓ L-theanine improves sleep quality by causing the brain to relax.[34] This is significant because many sleep-inducing supplements have sedative effects and can increase daytime drowsiness, a side effect not associated with l-theanine.[35]

Anti-Cancer Benefits

Green tea may play a role in preventing or managing oral, oesophageal, gastric, colorectal, bladder, ovarian, liver, lung, prostate and breast cancers.[36] This benefit comes from its antioxidants and anti-inflammatory compounds.

Please do not substitute your cancer treatment with green tea, though. Discuss with your doctors first, and if they agree, drink green tea as a supportive measure.

Heart-Protective Benefits

- ✓ Green tea may reduce LDL and total cholesterol levels.[37] When we eat, the liver secretes bile into the intestines to digest the fats in our food. To synthesize bile, the liver extracts cholesterol from the blood, reducing its levels. But, in the intestines, cholesterol is absorbed back into the blood along with digested fats. Green tea contains compounds that attach to this cholesterol in the gut and prevent its reabsorption. Consequently, this cholesterol is eliminated through the stool, effectively reducing blood cholesterol levels.[38]
- ✓ In cases of heart disease, oxidized LDL cholesterol lodges in the wall of the arteries, leading to plaque formation. The antioxidant activity of green tea can reduce this buildup.[39]
- ✓ Drinking green tea reduces the risk of heart disease.[40]
- ✓ When consumed in moderation, green tea has been shown to slow the progression of calcium buildup in the heart arteries.[41]
- ✓ Green tea reduces systolic blood pressure in patients with hypertension.[42] This effect is due to its catechins, which reduce inflammation and relax blood vessels (vasodilation), lowering blood pressure. Elevated blood pressure damages the inner lining of blood vessels, allowing the buildup of plaque. These narrowed arteries of the heart and brain consequently become highly susceptible to rupturing, triggering heart attacks and strokes. High levels of blood pressure can also harm the delicate filtration membranes in the kidneys, causing kidney damage.

- ✓ By reducing cholesterol and blood pressure levels – both risk factors for cardiovascular diseases – green tea helps lower the chances of heart attacks or strokes.[43] Truly a modern-day sanjeevani!

Anti-Diabetes Benefits

- ✓ Green tea has been shown to decrease fasting blood glucose and blood insulin levels.[44]
- ✓ It aids in lowering insulin resistance – where cells become less sensitive to insulin – one of the leading causes of type 2 diabetes. This reduces the risk of developing type 2 diabetes as well.[45]
- ✓ Green tea helps prevent certain diabetic complications through various mechanisms: boosting insulin activity, protecting insulin-producing cells in the pancreas, removing free radicals and alleviating inflammation.[46]

If you suffer from diabetes, drink green tea without adding any sugar or honey to it.

Anti-Obesity Benefits

There is some evidence that green tea may help you lose weight, contrary to this humorous quote found online.

> *'The only way to lose weight with green tea is to climb a mountain and gather the leaves yourself'*
> — UNKNOWN, social media

- ✓ Catechins can reduce body weight, body fat and waist and hip circumferences. They can also decrease visceral (belly fat deep inside your abdominal cavity on and around your vital organs) and subcutaneous (under the skin) fats.[47]
- ✓ Drinking green tea boosts the rate at which your body burns calories even when sitting idle (known as basal metabolic rate or BMR).[48] By raising your alertness and adrenaline levels, it also increases the expenditure of energy and promotes fat burning.[49]
- ✓ Caffeine enhances fat burning.[50]

Bone Health Benefits

- ✓ Green tea consumption reduces the risk of osteoporosis,[51] thanks to its antioxidants which keep the bones strong.
- ✓ A recent study involving post-menopausal women showed that those who had 1–3 cups of green tea a day were far less likely to develop osteoporosis than others who consumed less.[52]

We often associate bone weakness with deficiencies of calcium or vitamin D. But contemporary science recognizes that bones need more than just strengthening.

Under normal conditions, bones undergo a slow cycle of breakdown and rebuilding, with the balance between these two actions determining bone strength. The latter is dominant in youth while in ageing bones, their breakdown becomes a more critical factor, resulting in fragile bones or osteoporosis. Since inflammation accelerates bone disintegration,[53] the anti-inflammatory effects of green tea help protect against bone weakening.

Interestingly, many chronic inflammatory conditions completely unrelated to bones, such as obesity, type 2 diabetes, heart disease, memory loss, asthma and fatty liver disease, are almost always linked with bone loss[54] – signifying a link between systemic inflammation and bone degeneration. High body inflammation, therefore – coupled with low calcium intake and insufficient blood vitamin D – causes fragile bones, especially among elderly people.

Oral Health Benefits

There are specific harmful bacteria responsible for bad breath.[55] The catechins in green tea can destroy these bacteria effectively.[56] You may not want to carry green tea in a pouch for a quick swig before a date as there are better alternatives, but drinking it regularly can keep your mouth odour-free.

Joint Health Benefits

- ✓ The catechins in green tea offer support in osteoarthritis, a joint disorder in which the bone cartilage wears off.[57]
- ✓ It may alleviate symptoms of rheumatoid arthritis, a painful joint condition where the body's immune system mistakenly attacks the lining of joints.[58]

Since osteoarthritis and rheumatoid arthritis are inflammatory joint disorders, and green tea is known for its anti-inflammatory properties, they seem to be a perfect match!

Anti-Ageing Benefits

With its protective effects against so many degenerative diseases, why shouldn't green tea help us live longer! Recent scientific findings revealed that those who drank three or more cups of green tea per week had a much lower risk of dying prematurely compared to those who consumed less.[59]

Besides, green tea can also improve your quality of life due to its protective properties for your skin, joints and oral health. Was someone looking for the modern-day sanjeevani?

HOW TO CONSUME

The preparation of green tea is different from black tea.

How to Brew Green Tea

Take 250 ml of water. Heat it to about 85°C (185°F), short of bringing it to a boil. You should see bubbles now that are approximately 7–8 mm in diameter.

Add 2 g (1 tsp) of green tea leaves to the hot water. Let it steep for 3 minutes, before you strain and serve. Do not add sugar or milk to it, but a hint of honey or lemon can help enhance the flavour.

Note that green tea is a delicate brew. Do not brew it in boiling water (100°C) or it will turn bitter. On the other hand, the green tea leaves can be used multiple times, as they slowly release their beneficial compounds when brewed at around 85°C.

Some delicate varieties might require even lower temperatures, around 70°C (158°F). Always check the instructions on the packaging.

Chinese Method of Making Green Tea

The Chinese have a distinct way of preparing green tea. They first put the tea leaves in the pot and pour water heated to roughly 85°C (185°F) over them. After 30 seconds, they discard this water – a step called 'washing' the tea leaves, which removes dust or other contaminants from the harvesting and processing stages. Then they pour some more water over the 'washed' leaves, allow it to brew for 3 minutes and serve.[60]

Do you think we should also 'wash' black tea? After all, the same contaminants could tarnish black tea leaves too.

How to Brew Black Tea

Black tea is brewed differently. Firstly, water is brought to a boil at 100°C (212°F). Then, 2 g of black tea leaves are added to the hot water, and the heat is turned off. The brew is allowed to steep for 5 minutes before straining and serving. Optionally, sugar, milk, lemon, or cream can be added to taste. But remember to discard the leaves after brewing, as reusing them can lead to a bitter taste in subsequent brews.

Matcha Green Tea

Matcha leaves are even richer in caffeine and l-theanine. They are processed after removing their stems and veins. Then they are ground into a fine powder. To make matcha tea, pour water at approximately 70°C (158°F) over the powder, whisk it and consume. If desired, sugar or milk can be added to mask the tea's grassy taste. Because the leaves are consumed, matcha green tea is considered healthier than brewed green tea.

When Should You Drink

It's best to kick-start your day with green tea in the morning. As explained later, though, you are better off sipping small quantities of it throughout the day.
- ✓ Avoid drinking green tea at night because the caffeine in it may disturb your sleep.
- ✓ Try not to have green tea around mealtimes or when taking medicines, since it may prevent the absorption of some nutrients and medications. Keep at least an hour's gap, preferably two, in between.

A Case for Green Tea Supplements

Drinking green tea as and when you want can be challenging, especially when faced with a busy schedule, travel or social visits. Green tea extract supplements are a handy alternative in such situations, as they offer the same antioxidants. Opting for the decaffeinated variety of capsules allows for consumption at night without disturbing sleep patterns.

HOW TO SELECT

- ✓ Green tea should be green in colour! Some leaves may be brown or black if they are processed incorrectly.
- ✓ Here's a handy guide to the flavours of green tea leaves based on their colour:[61]
    - Dark green: Intense herbal notes

- Bright green: Herbal, but milder compared to dark green
- Greyish green: Bitter and astringent
- Olive green: Pleasant, with slightly sweet and toasty undertones

✓ Buy whole-leaf green teas. Tea bags are not ideal as they often contain small, broken tea leaf pieces called dusts, or fannings, which are left behind while producing high-quality tea leaves. When a tea leaf cracks, its essential tea oils start evaporating, reducing its aroma and smooth taste.

✓ Green tea leaves lose their nutrients and flavour over time. Consume within a year of production, independent of the expiry date on packaging.

✓ If you have access to harvest information (for instance, when you are visiting a tea plantation), choose tea leaves harvested in the first pick of the season (typically between April and May). These leaves have a better aroma and nutrients because during the dormant winter season, the leaves gather more natural sugars and have the least amount of astringent compounds called tannins.

✓ If you are concerned about potential pesticide and chemical contamination, choose organic green tea.

HOW TO STORE[62]

✓ **Odour:** Green tea has compounds that can absorb surrounding smells easily, so don't store it with any substance that gives off a strong odour.

✓ **Humidity:** The lower, the better. Above 70 per cent humidity, the leaves absorb moisture and develop mildew. To counteract this, use airtight containers.

- ✓ **Temperature:** Green tea's delicate compounds break down at higher temperatures. So, it should ideally be stored in the fridge to preserve its aroma and taste. Refrigerating green tea leaves can also extend their shelf life by six more months.

    Keep in mind that the container for daily use should not be stored in the fridge, as shifting it in and out can introduce moisture. Store bulk quantities in the refrigerator but keep a few days' worth of leaf supplies in a separate container outside.
- ✓ **Brightness:** Store tea in opaque containers as sunlight or artificial bright lights cause the compounds in green tea to oxidize.

How Much Should You Drink

Health benefits can be experienced from **three** cups (**750 ml**) of green tea consumed every day over several years. But remember, industry experts recommend dividing this quantity into **seven** to **ten small** cups a day. These small teacups are really popular (approximately **80 ml** each) in some East Asian countries. In India, this size is often called a 'cutting'.

Our body can absorb many nutrients in a limited quantity at a time. For example, your body struggles to mop up more than 250 mg of calcium in one go. Similar logic applies to the nutrients in green tea.

Ideally, adopt the wise Chinese approach: they serve small cups of green tea to guests. This way, they consume **80 ml** of green tea multiple times across the day, instead of drinking from one large pitcher (a practice often seen in the Instagram photos of many Indian influencers).

For Parkinson's disease: A standard 250 ml cup of green tea contains about 50 mg of EGCG, the most potent antioxidant catechin compound. Some significant research studies on Parkinson's disease involved doses of 300 to 500 mg of EGCG.[63] For this, you will need **six** to **ten** cups (**1,500–2,500 ml**) of green tea daily. This is a very high quantity to drink on a daily basis, potentially interfering with the absorption of other nutrients from your food. Also, this introduces 250–300 mg caffeine into the body, nearly two-thirds of the suggested daily upper limit on its consumption. One alternative, however, is to take decaffeinated green tea extract supplements. Since EGCG comprises half of the green tea extract, consume **600** to **1,000 mg** of green tea extract a day.

HOW MUCH IS TOO MUCH

- ✓ There are no toxicity studies on green tea.
- ✓ Overconsumption of caffeine from green tea can interfere with sleep and cause jitteriness, headaches or digestive problems.[64] The recommended upper limit for daily caffeine intake is 400 mg. This is equivalent to around **twelve** cups (**3,000 ml**) of green tea a day.
- ✓ If you are pregnant, there is a risk of preterm labour or miscarriage from excess caffeine. Do not exceed **200 mg** of caffeine a day in that case (**six** cups or **1,500 ml** of green tea).[65]

WHO SHOULD AVOID

- ✓ The catechins in green tea can hinder iron absorption in the intestines. So, drinking too much green tea can pose a risk of iron deficiency anaemia. Green tea can also interfere with the absorption of vitamin B_1, copper and chromium.[66] To sidestep these issues, don't drink it two hours before or after your meals.
- ✓ Cheaper varieties of green tea might be contaminated with heavy metals like aluminium or lead.[67] Stick to well-known, preferably organic, brands.
- ✓ Overconsumption of green tea can interfere with medicines such as statins for high cholesterol, beta-blockers for high blood pressure, chemotherapy drugs for cancer and specific antibiotics and antivirals for infections.[68] Maintain at least a two-hour gap between drinking green tea and taking these medications. While you may not be able to drink green tea in small cups at regular intervals because of such constraints, it will allow for the absorption of life-saving medicines.

SUMMARY

Systems and Benefits	Major	Minor
Anti-inflammatory	■	
Antioxidant	■	
Bones		■
Brain	■	
Cancer		■
Diabetes		■
Digestive		
Eyes		
Heart	■	
Immunity		
Joints		■
Liver		
Mental Health		■
Pregnancy & Lactation		
Reproductive		
Respiratory		
Skin & Hair		

Consumption: Drink **750 ml** a day, preferably divided over seven to ten times.

Excess: Avoid more than **3,000 ml** a day.

5

PAPAYA
Platelet Regulator

In the 1930s, Hawaii's booming papaya industry faced a devastating blow with the emergence of the papaya ringspot virus (PRSV), rendering the fruit inedible and causing a drastic decline in production.

As scientists sought solutions, they discovered the papaya's natural lack of resistance to the virus. Attempts at a technique called cross-protection, similar to human vaccination, failed.

Growing desperate, authorities commissioned a Hawaiian-born scientist from Cornell University, Dennis Gonsalves, to experiment with a genetically modified (GMO) version of papaya.

Altering plant DNA to cultivate more helpful traits underpins the entire premise of genetic engineering (GE), though its critics have long argued that if gone badly, these experiments can lead to 'Frankensteinian' foods.

In the 1990s, Gonsalves and his team conducted a groundbreaking experiment, implanting a gene from the virus into the genetic code of papaya, which fuelled opposition from critics of GMOs. Following this, a field trial was set up on the virus-devastated Puna island, where the new variety – 'Rainbow' – was planted alongside standard papayas. Within twenty-seven months, while regular trees were producing 2,000 kg of papayas per acre annually, the Rainbow variant yielded 50,000 kg.[1]

Today, the majority of the world's papaya crops are of the Rainbow variant – the only GMO fruit permitted in the US currently.[2]

Yet this history presents a profound ethical dilemma: should we forgo genetic engineering and let certain fruits and vegetables disappear? Or should we utilize it to rescue them? The next time you bite into a slice of papaya, remember that it represents a crucial aspect of the GMO food debate.

Papaya is a large fruit of the *Carica papaya*, a tall tropical herb with few branches. Originating in Central America, in 1550 it went to the Philippines with the Spanish before arriving in the Indian subcontinent. Today, it is grown in all tropical countries and used extensively in various cuisines worldwide.

NUTRIENTS

Papaya fruit has 88 per cent water, 11 per cent carbohydrates, 0.5 per cent proteins, and 0.3 per cent fats.[3]

Nutrition in Suggested Daily Amount of Papaya		Eat **150** grams
		Has **65** calories
Source	*Nutrient*	*Daily Need (%)*
Great	Vitamin C	116.3
	Vitamin B_9 (Folate)	28.5
Good	Magnesium	10.5
	Vitamin K	7.1
	Vitamin A equivalent	7.1
	Dietary Fibres	5.7
	Vitamin B_5 (Pantothenic Acid)	5.7
	Calcium	5.4
Poor	Phosphorous	4.9
	Vitamin E	4.5
	Copper	3.4
	Manganese	3.0
	Vitamin B_3 (niacin)	3.0
	Vitamin B_6 (pyridoxine), iron, vitamin B_2 (riboflavin), vitamin B_1 (thiamine), selenium, potassium, sodium and zinc	Less than 3

- ✓ As with most plant sources, papaya's vitamin A comes from antioxidant compounds called beta-carotenes.
- ✓ Some international studies have found high amounts of potassium in papayas.[4] The Indian research on local varieties, however, shows significantly lower amounts, making them a less reliable source.[5]

The papaya fruit has several nutritious plant compounds:[6]

- ✓ **Papain and Chymopapain:** Contain antioxidant, anti-inflammatory, anti-microbial, anti-clotting and protein-digesting properties.[7] They are present only in raw, not ripe, papayas.
- ✓ **Lycopene:** Antioxidant, anti-inflammatory, anti-cancer and anti-diabetes benefits and protects the heart, brain, bones, eyes and skin.[8]
- ✓ **Lutein and Zeaxanthin:** Antioxidant, anti-inflammatory and anti-cancer properties and protect the eyes, heart and brain[9]
- ✓ **Quercetin:**[10] Antioxidant,[11] anti-inflammatory,[12] anti-allergic,[13] anti-cancer,[14] along with brain-protective[15] and heart-protective properties[16]
- ✓ **Kaempferol:** Antioxidant, anti-inflammatory, anti-cancer and antimicrobial. It also protects the heart, brain, bones, liver, lungs and digestive system.[17]

The papaya leaves, but not the fruit, contain a fascinating plant compound:

- ✓ **Carpain:** It prevents low blood platelet count,[18] with anti-cancer, blood pressure-lowering and de-worming properties.[19] Later in this chapter, you will also see how carpain can help combat malaria and dengue fever.

HEALTH BENEFITS

Traditional Medicinal Uses

Various parts of the papaya tree are used in different treatments:[20]

- ✓ **Ripe papaya:** Ripe papayas can help alleviate chronic joint pain.
- ✓ **Unripe papaya:** Raw papaya is consumed for its laxative or diuretic benefits. It also stimulates breast milk production and induces labour or abortion in pregnancy.
- ✓ **Leaves:** They are used to treat malaria and smoked for asthma relief. A poultice of leaves is applied for nerve pain and on large swollen body areas in cases of elephantoid growth.
- ✓ **Juice:** The juice can be applied on warts, corns, tumours and thickening skin.
- ✓ **Seeds:** Papaya seeds are consumed to increase menstrual blood flow and expel intestinal worms. It is also used to abort a pregnancy.
- ✓ **Latex:** Fresh latex is applied to boils, warts, burns, freckles and psoriasis as an antiseptic. It is consumed to expel ringworms and roundworms, and can be applied to the cervix to contract the uterus, resulting in abortion.

Do remember that this information is intended to highlight certain ways in which papayas have been used over the centuries by practitioners of traditional medicine. Do not attempt any of them yourself.

Modern Medicinal Uses

- ✓ The papaya fruit exhibits antioxidant, anti-inflammatory, anti-cancer, heart-protective, brain-protective, anti-diabetes, digestive, respiratory and eye-protective benefits. It can also help heal gum disorders and infections.
- ✓ Papaya leaves contain antioxidant, anti-cancer, antibacterial

and immunity-boosting properties.[21] Since papaya leaves are not a part of our regular diet, they should be used for medicinal benefits only after a discussion with your doctor.

Antioxidant and Anti-inflammatory Benefits

Due to its antioxidant and anti-inflammatory compounds, consuming papaya can protect against many degenerative disorders, such as heart disease, cancer, diabetes, skin ageing, Alzheimer's disease, arthritis, cataract and other eye conditions.[22]

Heart-Protective Benefits

- ✓ The dietary fibre in papaya limits cholesterol absorption in the intestines, helping those who want to lower their cholesterol intake.
- ✓ Its anti-inflammatory compounds work against the inflammation-causing chemicals in heart arteries. This lowers the risk of heart disease, which can get aggravated by such chemicals.
- ✓ Antioxidants such as vitamin C and lycopene in papaya prevent the oxidation of fats, a process that initiates fat buildup in blood arteries.[23]
- ✓ The vitamin B_9 in papaya aids in reducing the risk of heart disease by converting homocysteine, a small protein (amino acid) in the blood, into other harmless proteins. Elevated homocysteine levels can increase cholesterol production and blood-clotting tendency.[24] They also raise oxidative stress, damage the inner linings of heart arteries and trigger heart blockages.[25]

Anti-Cancer Benefits

- ✓ Lycopene has been found to exhibit anti-cancer properties.[26] This can be especially helpful for someone undergoing radiation therapy, reducing the collateral damage caused by it.
- ✓ The beta-carotenes in papaya reduce the risk of prostate cancer.[27]
- ✓ Consuming papaya may help prevent stomach cancer.[28]
- ✓ It may also protect against breast cancer.[29]
- ✓ Papaya leaf juice has shown potential benefits against prostate cancer.[30]
- ✓ Papaya leaf juice can kill cancer cells in skin cancer (squamous cell carcinoma).[31]
- ✓ For diabetics facing an increased risk of liver, bladder, breast and prostate cancers, fermented papaya may lower blood glucose, reduce inflammation and control oxidative damage that triggers these cancers.[32] It is available as a food supplement, which is made from papaya fermented with yeast.[33]

As mentioned before, please continue with your prescribed cancer treatment and incorporate papayas into your diet only as a supportive measure after talking to your doctor.

Digestive Benefits

- ✓ Papain and chymopapain break down proteins in food, supporting digestion. These two enzymes are found only in raw papayas, but it's not advisable to eat uncooked raw papayas.

Wait, it gets worse. Cooking raw papayas actually destroys the two enzymes.[34] So the best solution is to consume them via digestive powders[35] or papaya leaf supplements[36] available in the market, which are made after removing any harmful substances.

✓ Papaya can provide relief to patients suffering from irritable bowel syndrome by alleviating constipation and bloating symptoms.

✓ The dietary fibres in papaya promote bowel movements.

Anti-Diabetes Benefits

✓ Oxidative stress significantly contributes to the development and progression of diabetes.[37] The antioxidant compounds in papaya protect against it, helping prevent or manage diabetes.[38]

✓ Papaya fibre reduces glucose absorption into the blood, preventing a surge in blood glucose levels after a meal.

✓ Papaya moderates post-meal blood glucose through additional mechanisms.[39] Some of its compounds stop certain digestive enzymes from converting the carbohydrates into glucose.[40] With less glucose available for absorption, the post-meal blood glucose spike remains regulated.

✓ Fermented papaya extract can decrease unhealthy chemicals in the bloodstream of type 2 diabetes patients.[41]

✓ Due to its sweetness, however, consume papaya in moderation, as excessive amounts may lead to elevated blood glucose levels. For those managing diabetes, it is recommended to keep portions small (**50 g**) at a time.

Brain-Protective Benefits

Fermented papaya powder has been found to reduce the chemicals that suggest oxidative damage in the brains of Alzheimer's patients in trials.[42] This kind of oxidative stress is considered one of the causes of Alzheimer's disease.

Eye-Protective Benefits

- ✓ The beta-carotenes in papaya help protect the cornea – the clear outer layer of the eye.[43]
- ✓ Vitamin C, beta-carotene, lutein and zeaxanthin can aid in preventing age-related cataracts in the eye lens.[44]
- ✓ Lutein, zeaxanthin and vitamin C can provide antioxidant support to the retina, protecting the eyes from age-related macular degeneration.[45]

Immunity-Protective Benefits

- ✓ The vitamin C in papaya boosts immunity.
- ✓ Its vitamin A content (beta-carotene) also plays a significant role in improving immunity.

Blood-Related Benefits

Papaya leaves can affect platelet count, which is important for blood clotting. Low platelet count can cause fatigue, bloody urine or stool, bleeding gums, easy bruising and longer bleeding from cuts.[46]

- ✓ In conditions like dengue fever, platelets clump together and get destroyed by the body's own defence system. To respond against the virus, your immune system creates chemicals (antibodies) that damage platelets further. The production of platelets also reduces in dengue fever. All this leads to a low platelet count, potentially causing internal bleeding or even death. Currently, there are no conventional medical treatments for it.[47] But papaya leaf extract can help:[48]

1. Prevent platelet loss through clumping[49]
2. Increase platelet production in the bone marrow[50]
3. Stop the dengue virus from replicating thanks to quercetin, an antioxidant

✓ The extract also increases platelet count in cases of other bleeding disorders.[51]
✓ It can be beneficial in treating malarial fever.[52]

Remember, these benefits come from papaya leaves, not the fruit. You'll find advice on the dosage later in this chapter. Some people prefer to make papaya leaf juice at home. A simple way to prepare it is also provided later.

Diseases like dengue, malaria and bleeding disorders need a doctor's care. Treating them yourself can be dangerous. Please always consult a doctor first.

Joint-Protective Benefits

The compounds papain and chymopapain in papaya latex, a milky liquid containing toxic compounds, reduce pain and inflammation in arthritis.[53]

Respiratory Benefits

✓ Beta-carotenes can decrease the chance of developing asthma.[54]

- ✓ Papaya alleviates asthma symptoms by reducing lung inflammation.[55]

HOW TO CONSUME

- ✓ Unripe papayas contain latex, a potent enzyme which is rendered safe for consumption upon heating. So, always cook unripe papaya.
- ✓ Allow an unripe papaya to ripen at room temperature for two or three days – as it ripens, the latex content decreases, making it safe to eat.
- ✓ Ripe papaya can be enjoyed raw, baked, stir-fried or puréed.
- ✓ Its flesh can be used to make papaya jam, smoothies, fruit salads and desserts.
- ✓ Papaya skin and seeds are edible but are often ignored. The crunchy, peppery tasting seeds can be rinsed with a strainer, air-dried and ground to a powder to be used as seasoning. They also offer many benefits of the papaya fruit.

How to Make Papaya Leaf Juice

- ✓ Cut the large leaf stems, leaving the small ones intact.
- ✓ Wash the leaves well to remove any dirt or droppings.
- ✓ Take 50 g of leaves, 50 ml of water and 25 g of sugar.
- ✓ Instead of sugar, you may use honey or jaggery to counteract the bitter taste.
- ✓ Chop the leaves into tiny pieces.
- ✓ Blend the mix until it turns into a deep-green liquid.
- ✓ Do not pass the liquid through a piece of cloth. Squeeze the pulp by hand to extract the juice before drinking.

If this sounds too time-consuming, you can simply buy bottled papaya leaf juice.

HOW TO SELECT

- ✓ An unripe papaya will typically exhibit a green or yellow skin, while a ripe one will have bright yellow-orange skin.
- ✓ Ripe papaya will feel firm to the touch, with no blemishes and emit a musky, sweet smell. The flesh inside should be orange, red or pink.
- ✓ Avoid ripe papaya that feels too soft and mushy, as its flesh tends to be bland in flavour.

HOW TO STORE

- ✓ Only store a papaya in the refrigerator once it's fully ripe.
- ✓ A ripe papaya can be kept in the refrigerator for up to a week to prevent further ripening. It's best to consume the fruit within two to three days.
- ✓ You can store a papaya in the freezer for up to nine months after removing the black seeds and cutting the fruit into small pieces.
- ✓ If you make papaya leaf juice at home, use it within a day. Store it in a sealed container in the fridge.

HOW MUCH TO CONSUME

- ✓ There's no set amount for daily papaya intake. However, a cup (**150 g**) per day is considered enough. Ideally, you should eat different fruits and vegetables on different days. Eating papaya three to four times a week is better than consuming it daily.

- In cases of dengue fever, it's advised to:[56]
  - Consume **30 ml** of papaya leaf juice three times a day before meals.
  - Start drinking the juice from the fever's onset.
  - Younger and older children should be given **5** and **10 ml**, respectively, thrice a day.
  - Don't expect immediate results; improvements should show from the second or third day.
  - Keep up the treatment until full recovery, even if symptoms improve.
  - Switch to papaya leaf extract tablets if your doctor advises to do so. Always consult your doctor before beginning any new regimen.
  - Dengue fever is a serious condition that requires immediate medical attention. Do not waste time trying any treatments on your own. Discuss taking papaya leaf juice or extract with your doctors and obtain their approval. Despite research published in prestigious international medical journals, many doctors may be unaware of this option.

HOW MUCH IS TOO MUCH

Don't eat more than **200 g** of papaya at once. Too much can upset your stomach and might even cause allergies in some individuals.

WHO SHOULD AVOID PAPAYA

- Pregnant women, because even a tiny amount of latex in unripe papaya can induce premature labour, causing uterine contractions and possibly abortion.[57] Ripe papaya is generally safe during pregnancy.

- Those allergic to latex, as papaya contains an enzyme called chitinase that can trigger an allergic reaction. This can turn severe and life-threatening, causing a condition called anaphylactic shock. The symptoms are swelling, nausea, vomiting, itching, wheezing, stuffy nose, dizziness, loss of consciousness and a drop in blood pressure.[58] Such individuals should also avoid drinking papaya leaf juice.
- Men seeking to start a family should steer clear of papaya seeds. They can affect sperm movement, which is crucial for fertility.[59] This effect is due to their alkaloid compounds that affect the male hormone testosterone and sperm activity.[60] Luckily, once seed consumption is stopped, this effect goes away.[61]
- Women who are trying to get pregnant should avoid papaya seeds, as they can affect the female hormone progesterone, preventing conception.[62]
- If you experience heart palpitation – a sensation that your heart is pounding or racing – especially if you are a woman above the age of sixty, it is best to avoid overconsuming papayas.[63]
- If you have been diagnosed with kidney stones, limit your papaya intake. Since it's high in vitamin C, the condition can potentially worsen.
- Though some websites argue that papayas can help lower elevated blood pressure levels because of their potassium content, the papaya varieties available in India cover just 2 per cent of your daily potassium needs.
- Those on diabetes medications should watch their papaya intake. It reduces blood glucose, which might lead to hypoglycaemia when combined with diabetes drugs.

SUMMARY

Systems and Benefits	Major	Minor
Anti-inflammatory	■	
Antioxidant	■	
Bones		
Brain		
Cancer	■	
Diabetes		■
Digestive	■	
Eyes	■	
Heart	■	
Immunity	■	
Joints		■
Liver		
Mental Health		
Pregnancy and Lactation		
Reproductive		
Respiratory		■
Skin & Hair		

Consumption: A cup (**150 g**) a day, three to four times a week.

Excess: Keep consumption below **200 g** a day.

6

SPINACH
Eye and Skin Guard

What comes to your mind when you hear the word 'spinach'? If your answer is 'iron', you may be a victim of a longstanding myth.

In 1870, German scientist Dr Erich von Wolf was researching the nutritional benefits of spinach. He recorded the iron content of spinach to be ten times higher than it actually was – misplacing the decimal point and noting 27 mg instead of 2.7 mg per 100 g of spinach.[1] This error went unnoticed for decades.

During the 1920s – a time of food shortages due to the First World War – America was battling its first malnutrition crisis among children. Authorities were urgently seeking a solution for iron deficiency and anaemia. Amidst the rapid development of nutritional science and mass media entered the perfect solution: Popeye.[2]

In 1929, cartoonist Elzie Segar created Popeye, a sailor who gained superhuman strength from consuming spinach. Due to the mistaken belief in spinach's unusually high iron content, government medical authorities decided to leverage Popeye's *popularity to promote spinach consumption. This campaign resulted in a 33 per cent increase in spinach sales across the US.*[3]

It wasn't until 1937 that scientists uncovered Dr Wolf's fraudulent or erroneous deed. By then, spinach had been marked as a superfood, and countless children were consuming it – inspired by their hero, Popeye – a glaring example of how mainstream culture can shape scientific beliefs.

Ninety years later, little has changed. Even today, doctors advise anaemic patients to consume spinach for its iron content, despite no scientific backing. While spinach does contain some iron, only about 5 per cent of it is absorbed by the body. Shockingly, you might find more iron in the dirt particles clinging to the spinach leaves rather than the plant itself![4]

But let's not blame Popeye entirely. The comic strip suggests that Popeye's strength is because of the vitamin A in spinach,[5] *not iron. Maybe Popeye knew that the only way to get iron from a can of spinach was to eat the can itself.*

Spinach (scientific name *Spinacia oleracea*) is a leafy green vegetable whose leaves can be enjoyed either raw or cooked. Its roots can be traced back to Persia nearly two millennia ago, where it was called *aspanakh*. In the seventh century, it journeyed to India, China and Nepal. At present, most of the world's spinach is produced in China and consumed worldwide.

NUTRIENTS

Raw spinach contains 91 per cent water, 3.6 per cent carbohydrates, 2.9 per cent proteins and 0.4 per cent fats.[6]

Nutrition in Suggested Daily Amount of **Spinach**		Eat **75 grams**
^		Has **17 calories**
Source	*Nutrient*	*Daily Need (%)*
Great	Vitamin K	658.6
	Vitamin B_9 (folate)	72.8
	Vitamin A equivalent	35.2
	Manganese	33.6
	Vitamin C	26.3
Good	Magnesium	19.8
	Vitamin E	15.2
	Potassium	8.9
	Vitamin B_2 (riboflavin)	8.9
	Calcium	7.4
	Vitamin B_6 (pyridoxine)	7.3
	Iron	7.0
	Phosphorous	6.1
Poor	Copper	4.9
	Vitamin B_1 (thiamine)	4.2
	Dietary Fibres	4.1
	Sodium	4.0
	Vitamin B_3 (niacin)	3.0
	Zinc, selenium and vitamin B_5 (pantothenic acid)	Less than 3

- ✓ Spinach contains a very high amount of vitamin K. Although the quantity is not considered dangerous, some people should avoid eating it, as we'll discuss later in this chapter.
- ✓ Even though spinach does not contain readymade vitamin A, the beta-carotenes in it are converted by the body into vitamin A. This is indicated in the nutrient table above as 'Vitamin A equivalent'.
- ✓ Here's the downside: anti-nutrients.[7] Despite being rich in iron and calcium, our body cannot absorb 95 per cent of these minerals due to the presence of compounds called oxalates in spinach. These oxalates bind tightly tightly to iron and calcium, preventing absorption in the intestines and reducing nutrient absorption in the body.[8]

Spinach also has plant compounds such as:
- ✓ **Quercetin:**[9] Contains antioxidant,[10] anti-inflammatory,[11] anti-allergic,[12] anti-cancer,[13] brain[14] and heart-protective properties[15]
- ✓ **Carotenes:** Antioxidant, anti-inflammatory, anti-cancer and anti-diabetes properties, and protect the eyes, skin, heart, brain and immunity[16]
- ✓ **Kaempferol:** Antioxidant, anti-inflammatory, anti-cancer and antimicrobial benefits and protects the heart, brain, bones, liver, lungs and digestive system[17]
- ✓ **Nitrates:** Protect heart health[18]
- ✓ **Lutein and Zeaxanthin:** Antioxidant, anti-inflammatory and anti-cancer properties, and protect the eyes, heart and brain.[19] Because they have similar structures, interchangeable in the body, they are collectively referred

to as lutein. Spinach is one of the best sources of both lutein and zeaxanthin.
- ✓ **Alpha-lipoic acid (ALA):** Antioxidant, anti-diabetes and anti-obesity properties[20]

HEALTH BENEFITS

Spinach can help maintain eye health, control blood pressure, protect against cancer and diabetes, make our bones stronger, and improve our skin, hair, blood and digestive health.

Eye-Protective Benefits

Let's first talk about how spinach can protect your eyes.

Lutein

Our bodies don't naturally produce lutein, the most potent antioxidant for the eyes. So it has to be obtained from food or dietary supplements. Once absorbed, it resides in the macula, the central part of the retina.[21]

Lutein has been extensively researched for its eye-protective features. However, there have been very few trials that specifically use spinach. The benefits listed below pertain to lutein. It's yet to be confirmed if spinach consumption lends similar benefits, although logically, it should.

Blue Ray Damage

- ✓ Blue and ultraviolet (UV) rays are known to cause eye damage. When these high-energy light waves come into contact with our eye cells, they dump their energy on them, causing light-induced oxidative stress. Regular exposure to these rays can damage or even destroy the eye cells without any antioxidant protection.[22]

- ✓ Lutein, being yellow in colour, absorbs about 90 per cent of blue light energy, thereby preventing oxidative stress and inflammation in eye cells.[23] As we age, the lutein levels in our eyes drop, making the cells more prone to damage and degeneration.

Age-related Macular Degeneration (AMD)

AMD is a condition characterized by a loss in the central field of sight. Studies suggest that increasing lutein intake can help protect against it.[24]

Diabetic Retinopathy

High blood sugar levels in diabetes can lead to diabetic retinopathy, a condition of the retina that causes vision loss. Lutein can protect the retina in such cases.[25]

Cataracts

When proteins in the eye lens turn opaque, they set off a condition known as cataracts, leading to blurry vision. Age-related cataracts are an outcome of lens degeneration triggered by oxidative stress.[26]

- ✓ Lutein is naturally present in the eye lens[27] and can reduce oxidative stress.[28]
- ✓ Eating more lutein-rich foods may decrease the chance of developing cataracts.[29] The more lutein you consume, the lower the likelihood of you developing cataracts.[30]
- ✓ Higher levels of lutein in your blood also correlate with a reduced risk of cataract.[31]

Will increasing your lutein intake now decrease the risk of cataracts, even if your past intake was low? The answer is yes.[32]

Glaucoma

Glaucoma is a common eye condition where the optic nerve connecting the eye to the brain gets damaged, causing vision loss. This occurs due to pressure buildup in the eye fluid.

Lutein can offer benefits for glaucoma patients.[33] But since glaucoma is like a plumbing issue in the eye – a mechanical problem – how can a nutrient be of any value here?

Well, it turns out oxidative stress can inflame and block the fluid drainage vents in the eye, increasing pressure buildup. As an antioxidant, lutein can help prevent or control this problem.[34]

A similar advantage for glaucoma will be highlighted in a later chapter about carrots, which are also rich in lutein. Please note that glaucoma demands immediate professional medical attention. While eating more spinach or consuming lutein supplements can't hurt, glaucoma shouldn't be self-treated as it could lead to blindness.

Dry Eyes

When eyes fail to produce enough quality tears for lubrication, damaging the eye surface and causing redness, burning and blurred vision, individuals experience dry eyes.

- ✓ Exposure to pollutants, ozone and ultraviolet rays can intensify oxidative stress and surface inflammation, resulting in dry eyes.[35]
- ✓ Lutein can help reduce the inflammation related to dry eyes[36] and, therefore, be deployed as a therapeutic treatment.[37]

Loss of Clear Vision

Our eyes weaken as we age, resulting in reduced sharpness (visual acuity) and less contrast in images (contrast sensitivity).

This can make activities like driving in poor weather more challenging. It also becomes difficult to discern dark objects against dark backgrounds – like a brown purse on a dark-coloured sofa – or bright objects against bright backgrounds, such as a white plate placed on a white tabletop. Activities where contrast provides crucial indicators to obstacles, such as climbing stairs or walking on potholed roads, become even harder to perform.

Moreover, some people can turn hypersensitive to glares or bright lights. When met with the headlights of an oncoming vehicle, they perceive only a blinding wall of white light. This intense glare results in visual fatigue, causing a delay in eye recovery.

- ✓ Lutein improves contrast sensitivity.[38]
- ✓ It can help with glare-induced disability and recovery time from strain induced by light.[39]
- ✓ It also improves visual sharpness and contrast in screen users.[40] Display screens have become an indispensable part of our lives: mobile phones, laptops, computer monitors, televisions, various digital consoles and so on. If you use any of these for several hours a day, regular consumption of lutein is vital. But how much should one consume? Stay tuned until the end of this chapter!

Heart-Protective Benefits

- Persistently high levels of blood pressure can damage internal organs. High blood pressure increases the risk of heart attacks, strokes and kidney damage.
- A diet high in potassium and low in sodium is essential for good cardiovascular health.[41] Scientists recommend that our potassium consumption be at least twice that of sodium. Our hunter-gatherer ancestors consumed sixteen times more potassium than sodium in their diets. But the potassium in our modern diet is barely three-fourths of the sodium we get from ultra-processed foods.[42] A low potassium intake can increase the risk of developing high blood pressure. As spinach is a good source of potassium, it can aid in lowering blood pressure and preventing high blood pressure problems.
- Spinach contains nitrates that boost nitric oxide (NO) in our blood vessels.[43] Nitric oxide helps relax vessel walls, reducing blood pressure.
- Rich in vitamin C, spinach helps the kidneys remove water and sodium from the body, resulting in lowered blood pressure.[44] It can also reduce blood pressure through other ways.[45]

Please do not alter your blood pressure medicines without professional advice. Incorporate spinach into your meals. After a few months, if your blood pressure improves, your doctor might consider lowering your medication dosage. This decision should always involve your doctors – never modify your medicines without their input.

Diabetes-Protective Benefits

✓ The leading cause of type 2 diabetes is insulin resistance, where the body cells are unable to utilize blood glucose even when there is insulin present. The nitrates in spinach help alleviate this condition.[46]
✓ Spinach increases post-meal satiety, reducing hunger pangs and cravings, and thereby curbing excess calorie consumption.[47]
✓ Alpha-lipoic acid (ALA) found in spinach improves fat metabolism and aids weight loss in obese patients. Since many people with diabetes often grapple with weight management issues, this can be especially beneficial for them.
✓ ALA also protects against diabetic neuropathy, a condition affecting those with long-standing diabetes and leads to nerve damage due to prolonged high blood glucose levels. Its main symptoms are pain and numbness in the hands and legs. Some people with diabetic neuropathy also experience problems with heart rate, bladder control and intestinal food movement. ALA is believed to mitigate diabetic neuropathy by preventing oxidative damage to nerves.[48]
✓ The dietary fibre in spinach can slow down the absorption of glucose from digested food, reducing the post-meal spike in blood glucose levels.

Cancer-Protective Benefits

✓ Eating a diet rich in green vegetables can lower the risk of developing cancer.[49]
✓ Spinach contains compounds that can help combat

cancers of the colon,[50] breast[51] and prostate[52] by preventing the mechanisms that lead to their development.[53]
✓ Its antioxidant compounds may help prevent and control cancer.[54]

However, please stick to your medical treatment for cancer. Talk to your doctor to see if consuming spinach can be a supportive addition.

Digestive Benefits

✓ Thanks to its high fibre content, spinach adds volume to meals and aids in preventing constipation.
✓ It also supports a healthy digestive tract by providing nourishment to gut bacteria. Although dietary fibres may not serve as a source of nutrition, they are essential for the intestinal bacteria living symbiotically within your body. Bear in mind that if these bacteria aren't healthy, your body's overall health will be compromised.

Bone-Protective Benefits

Spinach is a good source of calcium, but the presence of oxalates makes its absorption relatively poor. So, how does spinach contribute to bone strength?
✓ Spinach is rich in vitamin K, a crucial nutrient for bone health. Vitamin K enhances calcium deposition in bones.[55]
✓ It strengthens bone structure by helping produce specific bone-related proteins.[56]
✓ Unfortunately, even though vitamin K is densely packed within the fibrous mass in spinach, its absorption is

limited. A vitamin K supplement might offer up to 80 per cent absorption, whereas consuming uncooked spinach with a similar vitamin K content results in only around 5 to 10 per cent absorption.[57] Luckily, spinach contains an enormous amount of vitamin K, and its absorption increases by up to six times upon cooking.

Skin Health Benefits

- ✓ Spinach provides a significant amount of vitamin A, which helps produce collagen – a protein that maintains the skin's firmness and prevents wrinkles.
- ✓ Vitamin A prevents the skin from turning dry and flaky by promoting natural moisturizing, which aids in maintaining a youthful appearance.
- ✓ It also prevents acne.
- ✓ Spinach can help regulate the abnormal growth of skin cells, valuable in treating psoriasis and skin cancer.

We will discuss this more in the chapter on carrots.

Hair Health Benefits

Spinach helps in reducing hair loss in multiple ways:
- ✓ Its vitamin A content contributes to reducing hair loss.[58]
- ✓ Vitamins B and C accelerate the rate of hair growth and promote the production of proteins needed for healthy hair, collagen and keratin.
- ✓ Its antioxidants serve as protection against hair damage and loss due to pollution, heat and humidity, which cause oxidative stress.

Pregnancy and Lactation Benefits

✓ Spinach is rich in vitamin B_9, a nutrient required for the growth and development of the foetus.
✓ Pregnant women who incorporate lutein into their diets may find that their offspring exhibit better verbal intelligence and behavioural balance during ages six-and-a-half to eleven years.[59]
✓ When breastfeeding mothers consume lutein, it gets transferred to the infants via their milk,[60] fostering better vision and brain development.[61]

HOW TO CONSUME

✓ You can enjoy spinach raw in a salad or cook it as a leafy green side. Opting for the latter will render its nutrients more readily absorbable.
✓ Spinach pairs well with berries, eggs, nuts, citrus vegetables, pasta and fresh cheese. To add a kick of flavour to your spinach dishes, consider incorporating ingredients like ginger, garlic, chilies, cream or Indian spices.[62]

HOW TO SELECT

✓ Always buy fresh spinach. Look for vibrant green leaves and avoid any that are yellow, brown or wilted.
✓ Don't buy spinach if it is stored in a bag with excessive moisture.
✓ Ideally, spinach should be displayed in a temperature-controlled area of the produce section in a supermarket.

HOW TO STORE

- ✓ Remove any residual moisture from the leaves and place spinach in a plastic bag. For added freshness, wrap it in a paper towel before sealing the leaves in plastic.
- ✓ Do not wash spinach before storing it; rinse it just before use.
- ✓ Ideally, you should consume spinach within three days of harvesting it. While it can last up to a week in the refrigerator, some of its vital nutrients, like vitamin B_9, beta-carotenes and lutein, can gradually diminish over this period.[63]

HOW MUCH TO CONSUME

- ✓ There is no recommended 'dose' of spinach. Experts suggest consuming a cup (**75 g**) a day. But you don't need to eat it every day. In fact it is better to eat a variety of vegetables daily and include spinach every two to three days.
- ✓ You are advised to take **12 mg** of lutein (plus zeaxanthin) daily.
    1. A cup of raw spinach offers 9 mg of lutein.[64]
    2. If you are suffering from a medical condition that can be helped by lutein, eat around **20 mg** in a day.
    3. Consume **20 mg** every day also if you spend many hours staring at a screen.
    4. Lutein in fruits and vegetables is tightly bound within plant fibres. Cutting and cooking spinach releases it from these fibrous matrices, improving its absorption. How much? Various sources suggest this increase

ranges from minimal to almost doubling.[65] It is fair to say, though, that cooked spinach is likely more beneficial than its raw counterpart.
5. Lutein is a fat-soluble compound, better absorbed if consumed with fats. But since eating your spinach with a spoonful of oil would be too gross, enjoy it with a regular meal that includes some fats.
6. There are many other food sources of lutein, such as peas, corn, lettuce, kale, turnips, collards and even egg yolks. So, you don't have to rely solely on spinach to obtain your daily lutein.
7. Despite its availability in many foods, many people consume only about 1 to 2 mg of lutein a day.[66]

HOW MUCH IS TOO MUCH

✓ Daily spinach intake should not exceed **1 kg**, although it's unlikely that anyone, aside from perhaps Popeye, would consider consuming that much. There are four potential issues that may arise from consuming spinach in exceptionally high quantities:
  1. Spinach contains oxalates, which inhibit the absorption of essential minerals like calcium and iron.[67]
  2. Goitrogens, substances present in spinach that disrupt the production of thyroid hormones, can adversely affect thyroid function.
  3. Spinach's purine compounds can induce gout attacks.[68]
  4. The vitamin K in spinach can potentially cause blood-clotting issues.[69]

✓ Although the safe recommended daily level for lutein is **20 mg**,[70] no adverse side effects have been reported at much higher doses. Therefore, the risk of lutein toxicity does not directly decide the threshold for excessive spinach consumption.

WHO SHOULD AVOID

Eating spinach is usually safe for most people in regular quantities. But certain individuals might need to limit spinach consumption due to specific health conditions.

- ✓ If you're prone to kidney stones – formed when your urine has high concentrations of oxalates, phosphates, calcium or cysteine[71] – you might need to limit foods high in oxalates, such as spinach. A high intake of spinach can increase the risk of kidney stones.[72] If you repeatedly develop kidney stones, avoid eating spinach.
- ✓ Those with impaired kidney function should also limit spinach intake. Spinach has a high potassium content, which could worsen kidney issues in such individuals. If your kidneys are healthy, however, there's no need to worry.
- ✓ Spinach contains vitamin K, which aids in blood clotting, thereby counteracting the effects of blood-thinning medication.[73] Thus, if you're on such treatment, you should control your spinach intake.

SUMMARY

Systems and Benefits	Major	Minor
Anti-inflammatory		■
Antioxidant	■	
Bones		■
Brain		
Cancer		■
Diabetes	■	
Digestive		■
Eyes	■	
Heart	■	
Immunity		
Joints		
Liver		
Mental Health		
Pregnancy & Lactation		■
Reproductive		
Respiratory		
Skin & Hair		■

Consumption: Eat a cup (**75 g**) twice to thrice weekly.

Excess: Consuming more than **1 kg** daily can be dangerous.

7

GINGER
Digestive Dynamo

In 1928, a certain Mrs May Donoghue was at a cafe in Paisley, Scotland, enjoying a ginger beer, when she discovered a decomposed snail inside her bottle. Regrettably, she fell ill and later initiated legal proceedings against the ginger beer manufacturer, Mr Stevenson.

Before this incident, personal injury liability arose only upon physical contact with the victim. Therefore, if a manufacturer produced an unsafe product that caused harm, they were not held accountable.

In this particular case, however, the House of Lords – the Upper House of the UK Parliament – ruled the manufacturer at fault for neglecting to ensure the product's safety. This marked the first instance of negligence alone being sufficient cause for establishing liability.

The Donoghue vs Stevenson case[1] would become a landmark in the modern law of negligence. Strikingly, today's multibillion-dollar product liability lawsuits can trace their origins back to a single bottle of ginger beer.

Ginger, the stem of *Zingiber officinale*, is a plant commonly found in India, China, Australia, Africa and Jamaica. It belongs to the same plant family as turmeric and cardamom. Ginger's origins can be traced back to Asia nearly 5,000 years ago, and it holds the distinction of being the first spice traded with Europe. Today, this versatile root has found a global presence, not just in culinary practices, but also for its medicinal properties.

NUTRIENTS

Fresh ginger contains 79 per cent water, 18 per cent carbohydrates, 1.8 per cent proteins and 0.8 per cent fats.[2]

Nutrition in Suggested Daily Amount of **Ginger**		Eat **4** grams
		Has **3** calories
Source	*Nutrient*	*Daily Need (%)*
Poor	*All vitamins, minerals and dietary fibres*	Less than 3

While some sources suggest ginger has a substantial quantity of vitamin B_6, magnesium and manganese, this assertion is based on the consumption of 100 g of ginger in a day – an impractical, potentially toxic amount. The recommended daily intake is far less, around 4 g of fresh ginger, which will not provide significant amounts of vitamins, minerals or dietary fibres.

The medicinal benefits of ginger are derived primarily from its unique plant compounds:

✓ **Gingerols:** Contain antioxidant, anti-inflammatory, anti-

tumour, pain-killing, antimicrobial and liver-protective properties.[3] They are mainly found in fresh ginger.
- ✓ **Shogaols:** Antioxidant, anti-inflammatory and anti-cancer benefits.[4] They are present predominantly in dried ginger.
- ✓ **Paradols:** Antioxidant, anti-cancer, antimicrobial and anti-clotting effects[5]

HEALTH BENEFITS

Traditional Medicinal Uses

In both Ayurveda and Traditional Chinese medicine, fresh ginger and its dried powder form are considered distinct medicinal entities due to their differing properties. This difference arises during the drying process, as the gingerols in fresh ginger are converted to shogaols.[6] Interestingly, our ancestors found this out without the benefit of modern chemical analysis.
- ✓ In India, fresh ginger has traditionally been used for various ailments, such as cold, cough, colic, stomach upset, nausea, loss of appetite, asthma, heart palpitation, swelling and chronic joint pain.
- ✓ In China, the fresh root is used to alleviate cold, reduce nausea and detoxify the body. It induces sweating, thought to help get rid of infections.
- ✓ In China, dried ginger powder is used against 'cold' pain in the stomach, diarrhoea, cough and joint pain.

Indian medicine is grounded in the concept of *doshas* – *pitta*, *kapha* and *vata* – while Chinese medicine hinges on the principles of yin and yang. While they are both vastly different from modern Western medicine, it's really helpful to identify and examine what bridges these systems.

Modern Medicinal Benefits

Research from the last twenty years has revealed that ginger has antioxidant, anti-inflammatory, digestive, anti-diabetes, anti-cancer, anti-microbial, brain-protective, heart-protective and joint-protective benefits.[7]

One is left to wonder how traditional medicines discovered the benefits of ginger, which are similar to the ones identified through modern research techniques.

Antioxidant Benefits

Ginger contains compounds with strong antioxidant properties.[8] They protect against many degenerative disorders affecting the heart, brain, joints and eyes, as well as diabetes and cancer.

Digestive Benefits

- ✓ Ginger speeds up stomach emptying and aids in managing chronic indigestion, which occurs when the stomach takes too long to unload its contents into the intestines. While an occasional stomach upset could stem from overeating or food-borne pathogens, chronic indigestion is a systemic issue.
- ✓ It stimulates the movement of food through the intestines.[9] When food stays too long in the gut, the risk of gastrointestinal cancers increases.
- ✓ Ginger reduces nausea and vomiting experienced by pregnant women,[10] a condition commonly called morning

sickness, though it can occur at any time of day. The American College of Obstetricians and Gynecologists (ACOG) recommends using ginger capsules, candies, ale or tea for morning sickness as they can help soothe the stomach.[11]
- ✓ Ginger can also reduce nausea and vomiting induced by motion sickness or vertigo.

These benefits can be achieved by consuming **1 g** of dried ginger powder or **4 g** of fresh ginger daily.

Anti-Cancer Benefits

Gingerols, found in ginger, exhibit strong anti-cancer properties:[12]
- ✓ Gingerols reduce the colorectal cancer-causing toxic chemicals in the colon.[13]
- ✓ Ginger intervenes in processes that lead to various gastrointestinal cancers, including those affecting the oesophagus, gallbladder, liver, pancreas, stomach, small intestine, large intestine, rectum and anus.[14]
- ✓ Gingerols are toxic to the cancer cells, destroying them.[15]
- ✓ In cases of pancreatic cancer, ginger not only impedes the growth of cancer cells but also eliminates them.[16] It also helps against processes involved in the spread (metastasis) of pancreatic cancer.[17]
- ✓ Gingerols may help kill breast cancer cells and prevent their spread.[18] The shogaol compounds in dried ginger can prevent the growth of breast cancer tumours as well.[19]
- ✓ In ovarian cancer cases, ginger may induce death of the cancer cells.[20]
- ✓ Ginger can reduce nausea and vomiting induced by cancer chemotherapy treatments.[21]

Please note these findings are preliminary or resulting from laboratory studies. More clinical trials are needed to formally endorse ginger consumption as a treatment option. However, there's no harm in incorporating ginger into your diet after discussing it with your doctor.

Antimicrobial Benefits

- Ginger has compounds that combat many types of bacteria.[22]
- Some studies show that ginger extract can be used with antibiotics against certain bacteria.[23]
- Ginger oil has proven useful against bacteria found in throat infections in children.[24]
- Ginger extracts are beneficial against drug-resistant bacteria.[25] These are strains of bacteria that are difficult to kill with any antibiotic due to overuse of modern antibiotics.
- Gingerols in ginger kill bacteria causing gum disease in the mouth.[26]
- Ginger kills bacteria found in the lungs that cause various respiratory tract infections.[27]

You must, however, follow your doctor's treatment if you have a severe infection. Consuming ginger can maintain your immunity, thus possibly preventing such diseases.

Brain-Protective Benefits

Oxidative stress and neuroinflammation are believed to trigger or aggravate age-related brain degeneration, leading to conditions like Alzheimer's and Parkinson's diseases. Ginger –

with its antioxidant and anti-inflammatory properties – can help in the following ways:
- ✓ Prevent age-related brain decay[28]
- ✓ Potentially reduce neuroinflammation in the brain[29]
- ✓ Help prevent the blockage of blood supply in the brain[30]
- ✓ Possibly exert a protective effect against memory loss and Alzheimer's disease[31]
- ✓ May be utilized as part of a treatment regimen for Alzheimer's disease[32]

Please note that ginger has not yet proven to be a treatment for any of these conditions, though it has been used in traditional medicine for memory-related problems.

Anti-Diabetes Benefits

- ✓ Ginger slows down carbohydrate digestion,[33] reducing the amount of glucose produced from food for absorption in the gut.
- ✓ It enhances insulin secretion, which allows body cells to increase blood glucose utilization.[34]
- ✓ Ginger lowers insulin resistance[35] and may even help prevent it.
- ✓ Some compounds in ginger mimic insulin, promoting glucose entry into body cells.[36] In healthy individuals, insulin production is sufficient, so the benefit may not be significant. Ginger can help against insulin resistance, a common issue among diabetics.
- ✓ Does ginger help lower blood glucose? Many clinical trials have shown that ginger can reduce fasting blood glucose and average blood glucose, or glycated haemoglobin (HbA_1c).[37] Unfortunately, these trials were very short,

spanning eight to twelve weeks, making it difficult to measurably address diabetes, a condition that typically takes ten to fifteen years to develop. But these results are encouraging and indicate that ginger may offer benefits for blood glucose management.

- ✓ Ginger helps prevent or delay the onset of diabetes-induced medical complications.[38] Persistently high blood glucose levels can damage many organs, leading to heart disease, kidney damage, vision loss, bone and joint problems and dental and gum infections. Ginger can:
  1. Aid in preventing diabetic cataracts[39]
  2. Help protect against diabetes-related heart problems[40]
  3. Protect the liver, kidneys, eyes and neural system, the main organs damaged by diabetes[41]

Heart-Protective Benefits

- ✓ Ginger can reduce LDL cholesterol levels.[42]
- ✓ Some trials indicate that ginger can even reduce total cholesterol and blood triglycerides,[43] lowering the risk of heart disease.
- ✓ Ginger also decreases blood cholesterol by increasing the body's use of it.[44]
- ✓ It prevents processes that trigger inflammatory damage in blood vessels.[45]

Joint-Protective Benefits

Ginger relieves osteoarthritic pain and stiffness.[46] While osteoarthritis was previously considered a wear-and-tear problem of the joints, new research suggests that it is mainly an inflammatory condition, and ginger helps alleviate some symptoms through its anti-inflammatory compounds.

Obesity-Related Benefits

Ginger may also reduce obesity and body weight.[47] It can achieve this through multiple mechanisms:
- ✓ Reducing insulin resistance[48]
- ✓ Lowering inflammation in the body[49]
- ✓ Increasing the body's metabolic rate[50]

Women's Health Benefits

- ✓ Ginger is as powerful as certain pain relievers in easing dysmenorrhoea (painful menstrual periods),[51] which is possibly caused by chemical imbalances in the body.[52]
- ✓ Ginger can help reduce nausea during pregnancy.[53] But women in their third trimester should regulate their ginger consumption because too much of it may induce pre-term labour.

HOW TO CONSUME

- ✓ Raw ginger can be added to smoothies, salads, marinades, soups, gravies, curries, roasts and stews.
- ✓ Ginger can be baked in bread or biscuits.
- ✓ As a flavouring agent, it can be used with tea, beer, candies, gravies and meats.
- ✓ Ginger can be paired with spinach, chickpeas, lentils, carrots, meats, seafood and chocolate.[54]

Ginger can be consumed fresh or dried, as dried ginger powder, ginger preserve, crystalline ginger, ginger tea or water and ginger oil. Each of them has its benefits.[55]

- ✓ **Fresh Ginger:** Peel and slice or shred to use in cooking.
- ✓ **Dried Ginger:** Fresh ginger can be dried after peeling, with 4 g of fresh ginger yielding about 1 g of dried ginger. The dried form has a distinct aroma and flavour compared to fresh ginger.
- ✓ **Dried Ginger Powder:** Dried ginger is pulverized into fine particles. This releases its flavour and improves its texture.
- ✓ **Ginger Preserve in Syrup or Brine:** Immature green ginger can be preserved in sugar syrup or concentrated salt water (brine).
- ✓ **Crystallized Ginger:** Fresh ginger root is peeled, sliced and cooked in thick sugar syrup. It is then dried to create crunchy, sugar-coated ginger with a chewy centre. Coarse sugar is then sprinkled on top, which results in a tangy candy.
- ✓ **Ginger Tea:** Ginger 'tea' or ginger water, a more suitable phrase, does not involve tea leaves. It refers to steeping fresh ginger in hot water. Since it has no caffeine, it can also be consumed at night.

To make ginger tea, wash and grate 1 g (half a tsp) of fresh ginger. Leave the skin on, for most of the nutrients in ginger are just beneath its skin. Boil a cup (250 ml) of water and pour it over the grated ginger in a bowl (no more heating). Steep for ten minutes, strain and throw out the bulk. Flavour with honey or lemon juice, if desired. Add turmeric or black pepper to ginger for additional piquancy and nutrition.

- ✓ **Ginger Oil:** Commercial ginger oil is produced through steam distillation of fresh ginger or dried ginger powder. One kilogram of dry ginger powder will yield about 20 ml of extremely strong ginger oil.

    Since distilling ginger oil at home is difficult, here is an alternate method: mix 100 g of grated fresh ginger with 200 ml of olive oil. Bake the mixture inside an oven at 65°C (150°F) for two hours. Strain out the bulk from the clear oil.[56] This homemade oil will be a hundred times weaker than distilled ginger oil and up to 1 tsp (5 ml) of it can be eaten with food. Distilled ginger oil is too strong to consume directly.

HOW TO SELECT

- ✓ Choose ginger with a smooth, firm surface. If the skin is wrinkled, it is likely a dehydrated piece that has been lying around for some time. If the skin is soft or mushy, the ginger is spoilt.
- ✓ Ginger with mouldy skin or blemishes, or one revealing a brown or grey inner mass upon slicing, should be thrown away.

HOW TO STORE

- ✓ Ginger can be stored at room temperature for a week.
- ✓ To extend its shelf life to about three weeks, store ginger in a bag inside a refrigerator.
- ✓ For longer storage (up to three months), wrap ginger in plastic, place it in an airtight bag and store it in a deep freezer.

- ✓ Do not peel ginger unless you're ready to use it.
- ✓ Fresh ginger paste can last three to four months in the freezer.
- ✓ Pickled ginger can last up to three months in a refrigerator.
- ✓ Dried ginger powder can be stored for at least one year but loses its potency slowly over that period.
- ✓ Ginger tea can be refrigerated for a few days.
- ✓ Homemade ginger oil can be stored for up to six months.

HOW MUCH TO CONSUME

For better health, you can opt for one of the following: **2 tsp (4 g)** of fresh ginger, **½ tsp (1 g)** of dried ginger powder or **4 cups (1 l)** of ginger tea each day. It's a good idea to include ginger with your meals and aim to evenly divide your daily intake throughout the day.

HOW MUCH IS TOO MUCH

- ✓ Consumption of up to 4 g of fresh ginger daily is considered safe by the US Food and Drug Administration.[57]
- ✓ Clinical trials on ginger often use doses between 1,600 and 3,000 mg of dried ginger powder, equivalent to 6 to 12 g of fresh ginger. However, consuming more than 6 g of fresh ginger might lead to acid reflux, heartburn and diarrhoea.[58] Clinical trials are supervised by medical professionals, though. Without such guidance in normal life, it's safer to choose a smaller dose and take it over a longer period.
- ✓ Taking all of this into account, do not exceed either **6 g (3 tsp)** of fresh ginger, **1½ g (3/4 tsp)** of dried ginger powder, or **1½ l** of ginger tea a day.

WHO SHOULD AVOID

- ✓ Ginger helps increase the flow of bile from the liver. So people with gallstones should be careful in consuming excess ginger.
- ✓ Pregnant women should not consume more than **1 g** a day of fresh ginger or equivalent.
- ✓ Ginger should not be given to children under the age of two years.
- ✓ It can increase the risk of bleeding in people on blood-thinning medicines.
- ✓ Ginger can pose a risk of hypoglycaemia.
- ✓ It can reduce blood pressure. People who take blood-pressure-lowering medicines should watch out for very low blood pressure or irregular heartbeats.
- ✓ Do not eat too much ginger two weeks before and after any elective surgery to avoid chances of excess bleeding.

SUMMARY

Systems and Benefits	Major	Minor
Anti-inflammatory	■	
Antioxidant	■	
Bones		
Brain		■
Cancer	■	
Diabetes	■	
Digestive	■	
Eyes		
Heart		■
Immunity		■
Joints		■
Liver		
Mental Health		
Pregnancy & Lactation		■
Reproductive		
Respiratory		
Skin & Hair		

Consumption: **4 g** (**2 tsp**) of fresh ginger, **1 g** (**½ tsp**) of dried ginger powder (**½ tsp**) or **1 l** of ginger water a day, preferably in divided doses.

Excess: Avoid more than **6 g** of fresh ginger, **1½ g** of dried ginger powder or **1½ l** of ginger tea a day.

8

ALOE VERA
Skin Health Expert

In the world of celebrity endorsements, this story, a bit fictionalized, would stand unparalleled.

Picture ancient Egypt, circa 40 BCE. Archelaos, the marketing chief for the renowned Egyptian firm Nabtat Alkhulud ('plant of immortality'), which produces aloe cosmetics, excitedly announces to his CEO and board members, 'We've secured a huge celebrity endorsement for our creams. We need to change our ads, billboards, and even packaging.'

Philostratos, the CEO, is sceptical. He counters, 'Who can possibly be a better brand ambassador than the one we have had for the past 1,300 years – Queen Nefertiti herself?'

'No, we have someone else now,' the marketing head says, almost breathlessly.

'Who?' the board members ask, intrigued. After a dramatic pause, the marketing head reveals, 'Queen Cleopatra. She is using our products.'

Two of ancient Egypt's most beautiful queens and significant personalities, separated by 1,300 years, Queens Nefertiti (1370–1330 BCE) and Cleopatra (51–30 BCE), used aloe in their beauty regimens. Never before has there been a grander endorsement of an ingredient for skin health in history.

Aloe is a type of succulent that has been in use for thousands of years in many cultures around the world. It is thought to have originated in the Middle East. In Arabic, the word '*alloeh*', meaning 'shining bitter substance', perfectly describes its appearance and taste. Nowadays, it is cultivated in both tropical and arid regions worldwide.

There are at least 420 varieties of aloe, and aloe vera (scientific name *Aloe barbadensis miller*) is particularly popular. '*Vera*' in Latin means 'true'. In this chapter we will simply refer to aloe vera as aloe.

NUTRIENTS

The aloe plant consists of fleshy leaves, which are divided into three layers:
- ✓ The topmost layer, called the rind, is green in colour. It plays no role in our health.
- ✓ The middle layer contains a yellow-coloured latex. This has bitter laxative compounds.
- ✓ The inner layer, made up of translucent fleshy pulp, comprises around 96 to 98.5 per cent water. This pulp contains a viscous liquid called mucilage or gel, composed of 99.5 per cent water, and many valuable compounds but no laxative properties.[1]

Two Types of Aloe Juices

There are two types of aloe juices available in the market.

- ✓ **Gel Juice**: This juice is extracted solely from the inner gel of the aloe leaf. It has no laxative properties and is generally safe for consumption.
- ✓ **Whole-Leaf Juice**: This juice is extracted from all three layers of the aloe leaf, including the bitter latex. Consequently, it will have a purgative effect. Typically, such juice contains various toxic compounds from latex, which are filtered out by commercial manufacturers. Since the latex compounds are yellowish-brown, the filtered juice is called decolourized whole-leaf juice.

Nutrition in Suggested Daily Amount of **Aloe Vera Gel Juice**		Drink **80 ml**
		Has **12** calories
Source	*Nutrient*	*Daily Need (%)*
	Vitamin C	3.8
Poor	Calcium, iron, sodium, dietary fibres, vitamin A equivalent, vitamin B_1 (thiamine), vitamin B_2 (riboflavin), vitamin B_3 (niacin), vitamin B_5 (pantothenic acid), vitamin B_6 (pyridoxine), vitamin B_9 (folate), vitamin E, vitamin K, copper, magnesium, manganese, phosphorous, potassium, selenium and zinc	Less than 3

We'll primarily focus on the advantages of aloe gel juice, except when talking about skincare.

The pulp of aloe consists of 96.2 per cent water and 3.8 per cent carbohydrates.[2]

Aloe gel juice contains 99.5 per cent water and 0.5 per cent carbohydrates. Neither contains any proteins or fats.

Although aloe juice is not rich in vitamins and minerals, it contains a wide array of beneficial plant compounds, such as:[3]

- ✓ **Dietary Fibres:** Aloe contains minimal dietary fibres from a digestive point of view. But one of them is glucomannan, which offers many benefits even in small quantities. Glucomannans possess antioxidant, anti-cancer, immunity-regulating, wound-healing, bone-strengthening, neuroprotective and gut-health-promoting properties.[4]
- ✓ **Phytosterols:** These contain antioxidant,[5] anti-inflammatory,[6] anti-cancer,[7] immunity-supportive[8] and cholesterol-lowering properties[9].
- ✓ **Anthraquinones:** Found only in the latex of the plant, they irritate the inner lining of the intestines, increasing gut motility (peristalsis) and creating a laxative effect. Some anthraquinones also exhibit strong antioxidant, anti-inflammatory and antimicrobial properties.[10]

Besides these, aloe also contains a variety of antioxidant and anti-inflammatory compounds that protect against degenerative damage to various organs.[11]

HEALTH BENEFITS

Traditional Health Benefits

- ✓ **Ancient Egyptians:** Treating infections, for skin care and as a laxative.

- ✓ **Ancient Mesopotamians:** Gut-cleansing
- ✓ **Ancient Macedonians:** Healing wounds
- ✓ **Ancient Greeks:** Treating wounds, hair loss, genital ulcers and haemorrhoids.
- ✓ **Ancient Romans:** Treating wounds, digestive problems, hair loss, acne, sunburn, skin irritation and gingivitis.
- ✓ **Ancient Japanese:** Relieving sprains and aches
- ✓ **Native Americans:** Repelling insects
- ✓ **India:** Highly regarded in Ayurveda for digestion, beauty and skincare. It is referred to as 'ghrit kumari' in Sanskrit, meaning a young maiden, hinting that a woman should use aloe throughout her life to remain full of youth.

Modern Health Benefits

Aloe has anti-diabetes and anti-cancer properties and protective benefits for the skin, hair, digestion, immunity and oral health.[12]

It can be ingested orally or applied topically, with each method imparting its own advantages. We will focus primarily on the beneficial effects of consuming aloe juice.

Digestive Benefits

- ✓ Aloe juice can ease symptoms of acidity without the adverse effects associated with antacids.
- ✓ With a water composition of 99.5 per cent, aloe juice elevates the volume of fluids in the gastrointestinal tract.
- ✓ It stimulates mucus secretion and promotes movement of food in the intestines.[13]
- ✓ Strong laxative compounds in aloe vera reach the colon undigested, leading to the production of softer stools. This

characteristic is specifically linked to whole-leaf juice.
- ✓ Aloe can soothe symptoms of irritable bowel syndrome.[14]

Anti-Diabetes Benefits[15]

- ✓ Aloe prevents glucose absorption in the intestines, lowering post-meal blood glucose levels.[16]
- ✓ It increases insulin sensitivity, the body's ability to utilize insulin from blood glucose,[17] lowering the risk of type 2 diabetes.
- ✓ By improving insulin sensitivity, aloe reduces fasting blood glucose in pre-diabetics (a step before a person develops diabetes).[18]
- ✓ Aloe has been found to reduce average blood glucose (HbA_1c) in people with type 2 diabetes after a few months of use.[19]
- ✓ It may reduce blood pressure and cholesterol in type 2 diabetics.[20]
- ✓ It also exhibits fewer side effects compared to diabetes medicines.[21]

Skin-Protective Benefits

Aloe is well-known for its skin-health benefits and ability to repair damaged skin, particularly when applied topically as a gel. While the chapter on carrots explains how vitamin A helps our skin stay healthy by fortifying its structural strength, aloe 'rebuilds' the skin after it has broken down.

The effects of aloe and vitamin A on the skin are similar. But each presents a few advantages that the other does not.

Wound Healing[22]

- ✓ Aloe gel reduces inflammation around wound sites.[23]

- ✓ It prevents the creation of histamines, substances that cause skin irritation and itching.
- ✓ It enhances the immune system activity needed for wound healing.[24]
- ✓ Aloe accelerates healing by increasing collagen cross-linking in the wound.[25] This cross-linkage functions similarly to the stitches used in darning, which is the process of repairing a torn piece of fabric.
- ✓ Aloe gel hydrates and protects the skin from dryness and cracking.
- ✓ Glucomannans promote collagen production, improve skin health, increase moisture, reduce redness and prevent ulcers.[26]
- ✓ It contains zinc, an astringent that helps woundsites heal by tightening them.
- ✓ Aloe increases the strength of scar tissue by improving collagen activity and promoting wound contraction.[27]

Skin Inflammation

It blocks the production of an inflammatory substance, prostaglandin E_2, in the skin.[28] This reduces inflammation and redness.[29]

Skin Ulcer

Many studies have demonstrated the effectiveness of aloe in treating diabetic wounds, ulcers, bedsores and mouth sores.[30]

Sunburn

- ✓ Application of aloe gel can soothe sunburnt skin.
- ✓ Its anti-inflammatory compounds help reduce skin redness.

- ✓ The glucomannans have regenerative properties that aid in healing sunburn.[31]
- ✓ Aloe can help with first-degree (superficial) and second-degree (blistering) sunburns.[32]
- ✓ Thanks to its phytosterol content, daily oral consumption of aloe can boost the strength, moisture and elasticity of sunburnt skin.[33]

Skin Ageing

Aloe tightens the skin and reduces wrinkles, which slows the ageing process. When applied to the skin, it exhibits the following properties:

- ✓ Aloe hydrates dry skin due to its glucomannan compounds.
- ✓ It causes skin cells to stick together, reducing flaking and thus leading to smoother skin.
- ✓ Aloe's amino acids soften tough skin cells, resulting in more youthful and vibrant skin.
- ✓ It stimulates skin cells to produce collagen (skin-firming protein) and elastin (skin elasticity-enhancing protein).
- ✓ It contains zinc, which, as mentioned earlier, tightens skin pores through its astringent action.

Acne

When exposed to toxins or pathogens, the skin produces a substance that causes inflammation.[34] This stimulates oil-secreting glands in the skin to go into overdrive and produce more oil, leading to acne.[35] Aloe reduces the production of the inflammatory chemical, thus controlling acne outbreaks.[36]

Eczema

Aloe's anti-inflammatory properties make it effective at preventing eczema flare-ups, which are inflammatory skin reactions.[37]

Psoriasis

The National Psoriasis Foundation recommends applying a 0.5 per cent aloe cream to psoriasis-affected skin three times per day to help reduce redness and scaling.

Dandruff

Dandruff is caused by the presence of malassezia, a fungus that lives on our scalps in a mutually beneficial relationship. It competes with other pathogens for the same nutrients, preventing them from growing on our scalps. The fungus feeds on the oil produced by the scalp skin and excretes oleic acid. If the fungus grows too much, excess oleic acid is produced, which may penetrate the top layer of the scalp skin. This may cause an allergic reaction in people who are sensitive to oleic acid. Their scalp starts shedding its uppermost layer to quickly eliminate the irritant. The resulting skin flakes are dandruff.

Aloe controls dandruff by alleviating fungal infection, excess inflammation and flaky skin when applied to the scalp.[38]

Hair-Protective Benefits

Aloe can promote new hair growth by increasing blood circulation to the scalp and breaking down proteins in dead cells.

Immunity-Protective Benefits

Aloe contains numerous antiseptic compounds that prevent viral, bacterial and fungal infections.[39] These compounds inactivate a variety of viruses, including influenza, herpes simplex[40] and varicella zoster.[41] Applying aloe gel to the affected skin may help combat these infections.

Cancer-Protective Benefits

- ✓ Aloe has shown promise in clinical trials as an early-stage protection against cancers of the breast,[42] pancreas[43] and skin[44]. Scientists have attributed these benefits to compounds such as emodin and aloe-emodin.
- ✓ It inhibits the growth of human breast and cervical cancer cells.[45]
- ✓ Additionally, aloe has been found to inhibit cancer progression through at least ten different mechanisms, including:[46]
    1. creating an environment to reduce the chances of tumour growth[47]
    2. increasing antioxidant activities that force tumour cells to kill themselves (autophagy)
    3. glucomannan compounds preventing tumour cells from spreading to other regions (metastasis)

Please do not substitute aloe for cancer treatment because these findings are all preliminary. They do, however, suggest that aloe may have a lot of undiscovered cancer-fighting benefits.

Oral Health Benefits

Aloe reduces dental plaque and gingivitis, a gum disease that causes irritation, redness and swelling at the base of teeth.[48]

HOW TO CONSUME

How to Select Aloe Leaves

Many people prefer to grow aloe plants themselves, while others prefer to buy the leaves.
- ✓ When harvesting leaves, select mature plants in the ground.
- ✓ Look for leaves with rosy-pink tips, indicating ripeness.
- ✓ Select plump, fleshy leaves in the upper part of the plant. Avoid wrinkled, limp or small leaves near the plant's base.

How to Prepare Aloe Gel Juice

- ✓ Don't pull out the leaves from a plant; instead, use a sharp knife or scissors to cut them close to the trunk.
- ✓ Place the leaves in a glass with the cut side down to let the toxic yellow latex drain out. It can be harmful in large amounts and cause diarrhoea or allergies in some people.
- ✓ Once drained, trim off the spiky edges. Then slice out the skin to extract the clear white gel from inside. Throw away the green skin and any yellow latex.
- ✓ Juice this gel on its own or mix it with fruits or blend it with vegetables.
- ✓ Do not try to prepare aloe whole-leaf juice at home due to toxicity concerns.

How to Select Aloe Products

- ✓ Choose between aloe gel juice and aloe whole-leaf juice available at stores. Since the latex contains bitter and

laxative anthraquinone compounds that are toxic in higher concentrations, the manufacturers typically remove them by a filtration process called decolourization, making the juice safe for daily consumption.
- ✓ Be aware that some manufacturers may not completely remove these bitter compounds, instead diluting them by adding sugar and flavours. These added sugars can make the juice less healthy, so read the label carefully.
- ✓ Aloe labelling may be inconsistent or incorrect since making aloe juices and gels is almost a cottage industry. Look for a well-known, trusted brand.
- ✓ Because aloe gel consists of 99.5 per cent water, the cream version is available as a 0.5 per cent gel.[49] Some manufacturers concentrate the gel further to get 1 per cent gel.
- ✓ For specific treatments like psoriasis, the gels can include higher concentrations of aloe solids, reaching up to 70 per cent aloe solids (with 30 per cent water).

HOW TO STORE

- ✓ The gel extracted at home can be stored in a refrigerator for two weeks if kept in an airtight container. If you opt for freezing, it can last for up to a year in a deep freezer.
- ✓ Once you've opened a bottle of aloe juice, it should be refrigerated. If the juice is preservative-free, use it within thirty days of opening. You can add four more months to its life if it includes preservatives.[50]

HOW MUCH TO CONSUME

- ✓ There are no recommended guidelines for aloe consumption at present.

- ✓ Experts generally suggest drinking as many millilitres of pure 100 per cent aloe gel juice as your body weight in kilograms. If you weigh 80 kg, you should take **80 ml** daily. Keep in mind that aloe gel juice is 99.5 per cent water. So, 80 ml will contain about 400 mg of aloe solids, with the remainder being water.
- ✓ Many aloe trials have used 500 mg of aloe ingredients daily, indicating that the suggested juice quantity is in that range.
- ✓ If the juice is diluted, adjust your consumption to get the equivalent amount of aloe compounds. For example, if the liquid is 80 per cent pure, consume 100 ml of it instead of 80 ml of 100 per cent pure juice.
- ✓ Obviously, if you purchase a 10 per cent pure juice bottle, drinking 800 ml daily would be a punishment. In such cases, simply buy a different product.
- ✓ Some authoritative sources suggest drinking 250 ml (one glass) of aloe juice daily.[51] But in my opinion, this is excessive for most people to drink without developing digestive issues, unless the experts are referring to a highly diluted, 30 per cent or less pure, version.
- ✓ For blood glucose control, aim for a daily intake of **300 mg** aloe compounds.[52] Adjust your juice intake depending on its potency.
- ✓ To improve cholesterol and triglyceride levels, take **500 mg** of aloe compounds twice a day. Keep in mind that this is a high dosage, almost equivalent to **200 ml** of pure aloe juice.
- ✓ For benefits related to diabetes, it's best to take aloe with meals. But for digestive benefits, it's better consumed on an empty stomach.

HOW MUCH IS TOO MUCH[53]

- ✓ Aloe gel juice is usually considered safe, but don't drink more than **250 ml** every day as this can cause stomach upset or diarrhoea.
- ✓ If you prefer whole-leaf juice, it's important to be cautious. Check for a harmful substance called aloin, which can sometimes mix with the juice from the latex part of the aloe.[54] The industry standard, though not regulated, is not to exceed ten parts per million (PPM) aloin in such juice, meaning the juice should have less than 10 mg of aloin per litre.[55] Unfiltered whole-leaf juice has at least 200 mg – often much more – of aloin per litre, an unsafe quantity for drinking. Some manufacturers filter out the aloin, leaving behind decolourized whole-leaf juice, which is safe to drink. But if the juice is not filtered enough, you run the risk of aloin toxicity. As labels in the aloe industry can sometimes be inaccurate, it's better to drink less than **50 ml** of any aloe whole-leaf juice per day.
- ✓ If you extract whole-leaf juice at home, it may contain toxic levels of aloin, which is why it is best to avoid homemade whole-leaf juice. Instead, consume home-made aloe gel juice as it won't contain aloin.
- ✓ Some people might experience an upset stomach when they first start drinking aloe juice. To prevent this, try splitting your daily amount into two or three smaller servings and gradually increasing how much you drink. Starting with a small amount like 30 ml and monitoring how your stomach reacts is a smart approach.

- ✓ It should be obvious, but aloe gels intended for skin application should never be ingested!

WHO SHOULD AVOID

- ✓ Be careful when using aloe with diabetes medicines. Together, they may cause hypoglycaemia. Symptoms include fatigue, sweating, an irregular heart rhythm, blurred vision, confusion and loss of consciousness. Before incorporating aloe in your diet, consult your doctor if you are on anti-diabetes medicines.
- ✓ Pregnant women should not take aloe orally, as it can cause uterine contractions and possibly miscarriage.[56]
- ✓ Aloe consumption while breastfeeding may cause stomach upset in the infant. As aloe's other effects on babies are not clear, nursing mothers should avoid it.[57]
- ✓ Children under twelve years of age should not drink aloe latex or whole-leaf extracts, even if their bitter compounds are removed.
- ✓ The latex in aloe is known to interact with many common medicines, including blood thinners, diuretics, diabetes medicines and laxatives.[58] If you are on any of these medications, avoid consuming whole-leaf aloe juice.
- ✓ As of now, there is no scientific evidence supporting the claim that anthraquinones in aloe cause colorectal cancer.[59]

SUMMARY

Systems and Benefits	Major	Minor
Anti-inflammatory	■	
Antioxidant	■	
Bones		
Brain		
Cancer		■
Diabetes	■	
Digestive	■	
Eyes		
Heart		
Immunity		■
Joints		
Liver		
Mental Health		
Pregnancy & Lactation		
Reproductive		
Respiratory		
Skin & Hair	■	

Consumption: 1 ml of a hundred per cent pure aloe gel juice per kg of body weight, divided over two to three doses daily.

Excess: Avoid more than **250 ml** of aloe gel juice or **50 ml** of decolourized whole-leaf juice daily.

9

TURMERIC
Liver Protector

Turmeric, known as 'haldi' in Hindi, holds immense significance in Hindu traditions, symbolizing inner purity and auspicious beginnings.[1]

In Hindu weddings, the application of turmeric signifies an auspicious start to the marriage rituals. Even some wedding invitation cards are marked with turmeric before being sent to guests.

A ceremony called 'haldi' marks the start of the rituals. The bride and the groom are anointed with a paste made from turmeric in their respective homes, signifying the purification of mind and body before the wedding. Turmeric is applied to their faces, not only to lighten the skin but also to lend it a glow and calm the couple's nerves.[2]

Furthermore, turmeric symbolizes prosperity. The groom and the bride wear yellow clothes (traditionally dyed with turmeric) to invite peace and affluence into their married life. Any piece of clothing tinted with turmeric signifies protection from illnesses.

Turmeric also symbolizes fertility. During the wedding ceremony, the groom ties a string soaked in turmeric paste around the bride's neck, indicating the woman's now married status. This amulet, known as the mangalsutra, is said to offer her protection and good health.[3]

Hindu weddings are rarely considered complete without the presence of turmeric.[4]

Turmeric (scientific name *Curcuma longa*) is a plant related to the ginger family. It was initially used as a dye for the robes of priests but, over time, turmeric became a popular spice in South Asian cuisines. Known for its pungent flavour with a mild ginger or orange-like aroma, it lends South Asian curries their traditional bright-yellow colour. Moreover, turmeric has been a staple in traditional medicinal systems, such as Ayurveda, traditional Chinese medicine, and the Unani and Siddha practices.[5]

NUTRIENTS

Turmeric contains 13 per cent water, 67 per cent carbohydrates, 9.6 per cent proteins and 3.3 per cent fats.[6]

Nutrition in Suggested Daily Amount of Turmeric		Eat **6** grams
		Has **19** calories
Source	*Nutrient*	*Daily Need (%)*
Great	*Manganese*	59.4
Good	*Iron*	11.4
	Magnesium	4.2
	Copper	3.9
	Dietary Fibres	3.4
	Phosphorous	3.0
Poor	*Vitamin E, potassium, zinc, vitamin K, calcium, selenium, vitamin B_5 (pantothenic acid), vitamin B_9 (folate), vitamin B_2 (riboflavin), vitamin B_3 (niacin), vitamin B_6 (pyridoxine), vitamin B_1 (thiamine), sodium, vitamin C and vitamin A equivalent*	Less than 3

Some websites claim that turmeric is an excellent source of dietary fibre and omega-3 fatty acids.[7] But this assertion is impossible since typical daily consumption is only around 6 g.

Turmeric contains healthy plant chemicals known as curcuminoids.[8] The primary curcuminoid among them, making up around 80 per cent, is a compound called curcumin. Since other curcuminoids share similar structures and benefits with curcumin, the collective term 'curcumin' is often used to refer to the entire group.

HEALTH BENEFITS

Traditional Medicinal Uses

- ✓ In Ayurveda, turmeric is revered for its healing properties against liver disorders, rheumatism and respiratory conditions such as asthma, allergies, cough and sinusitis. It also addresses health issues like arthritis, diabetic wounds, sprains and swellings. Turmeric boosts energy levels, improves digestion, reduces flatulence, eliminates intestinal worms, purifies the blood and regulates menstruation. It also serves as an antiseptic and antibacterial remedy for cuts and burns and, when applied topically, can treat skin conditions.
- ✓ In Traditional Chinese medicine, turmeric is considered to be a herb that invigorates the blood.[9] It is used to improve circulation in cases of cardiovascular disorders and menstrual irregularities, to alleviate acute pain and address tumours and clots caused by blood stagnation.
- ✓ In Unani medicine, turmeric is used to dilate blood vessels, promoting better blood circulation. It is also used to expel phlegm.

Many of the health benefits attributed to turmeric by modern science are similar to those recognized in tradition medicine, reminding us of the wisdom inherent in our ancestral knowledge.

Modern Medicinal Uses

Curcumin and turmeric have been extensively studied in recent decades. Curcumin exhibits powerful antioxidant and anti-inflammatory properties. Most of its other benefits spring from these qualities, including its anti-cancer, anti-diabetes, heart-protective, liver-protective, brain-protective, antimicrobial and digestive properties.[10] These functions prove the vital role antioxidants and anti-inflammatory compounds play in protecting against heart disease, memory loss, diabetes, cancers, fragile bones, joint pain and age-related eye disorders.

Antioxidant Benefits

- ✓ Turmeric exhibits strong antioxidant properties.[11]
- ✓ Curcumin can prevent free radical damage and lower the risk of many degenerative disorders.[12]
- ✓ It also elevates the function of internally produced antioxidants in our bodies, called endogenous antioxidants, yielding a dual benefit.[13] This amplifies the antioxidant effect of turmeric.[14]

Anti-inflammatory Benefits

Turmeric possesses anti-inflammatory properties that can reduce inflammatory processes and chemicals in the body.[15] It can also be used to treat various inflammatory disorders.[16]

Anti-Cancer Benefits

Curcumin and turmeric protect against many aspects of cancer:[17]

- ✓ **Cell damage:** Curcumin prevents the replication of genetically damaged cells.[18] When a cell's DNA is compromised, it can grow unrestrained, resulting in or worsening cancer.
- ✓ **Cell growth:** Curcumin regulates a critical process in cell growth, known as differentiation.[19] If a cluster of cells

grows without undergoing this process, it can develop into a tumour.
- ✓ **Blood supply:** Curcumin blocks new blood vessel development that cancer cells rely on, slowing their rapid growth.[20] As cancer tumours grow larger than a few millimetres, the regular blood supply can no longer meet their nutrient requirements. So, they secrete chemicals to trigger the growth of new blood vessels (neoangiogenesis), thereby providing more blood and nutrients.
- ✓ **Cancer spread:** Curcumin prevents cancer cells from spreading to new locations in the body.[21] During a certain stage of tumour growth, some cancer cells can move away from their original location, causing the cancer to spread (metastasis).

However, turmeric is not a remedy for cancer. If you are undergoing cancer treatment, you must continue taking your prescribed medicines. Consult your doctor if you want to add turmeric to your diet as a supportive measure.

Liver-Protective Benefits

Certain medications, alcohol, toxic chemicals in the air and water, malaria parasites, dengue or chikungunya viruses and poor dietary habits can all cause liver damage. Long-term harm can result in fatty liver (NASH and NAFLD), liver fibrosis, cirrhosis and, eventually, liver cancer.
- ✓ Curcumin can protect against liver problems.[22]
- ✓ It can lower blood chemical levels related to liver diseases, such as alkaline phosphatase, SGOT (or AST) and SGPT (or ALT).[23]
- ✓ Curcumin boosts the liver's natural protective antioxidant levels.[24]

- ✓ It prevents alcohol-induced liver fibrosis.[25]
- ✓ In case of liver sepsis, curcumin can alleviate severe liver inflammation and prevent liver failure.[26] When the liver is damaged by pathogens or toxins, certain harmful inflammatory chemicals are produced. These, collectively, cause the cells to function improperly, leading to liver sepsis and failure thereafter. Please note that liver sepsis is a life-threatening medical emergency that requires immediate medical help. This point is just to highlight the capabilities of curcumin.

Brain-Protective Benefits

Chronic brain inflammation can lead to the degradation and death of brain cells. Alzheimer's disease, Parkinson's disease, depression and epilepsy have all been linked to neuroinflammation.[27] The green tea chapter contains additional insights on brain degeneration.

- ✓ While most antioxidants cannot cross the BBB, curcumin can penetrate this layer and help brain cells by acting as an antioxidant, anti-inflammatory and anti-protein-accumulation agent.[28] It may even be able to prevent or control neurodegenerative disorders.[29]
- ✓ Turmeric may prevent Alzheimer's and depression through another mechanism. Curcumin can increase the levels of a protein in the brain known as brain-derived neurotrophic factor (BDNF), which promotes nerve cell growth and maintenance while also improving their connectivity, essential for learning and memory.[30] Reduced BDNF protein levels have been observed in brain disorders such as Alzheimer's disease and depression.[31]

- ✓ Curcumin has been linked to increased levels of docosahexaenoic acid (DHA) – an omega-3 fatty acid that promotes brain health.[32] For people who do not consume fish oil on a regular basis, this may protect them from a variety of brain disorders.

Mental Health Benefits

- ✓ Curcumin has been found to be as effective as antidepressant medicines in treating depression.[33]
- ✓ In individuals with obesity, curcumin can alleviate symptoms of anxiety and depression.[34]
- ✓ Chronic stress can impair the brain's learning abilities. Curcumin has been found to reverse such damage,[35] mirroring the effects of an antidepressant medicine called imipramine.

Heart-Protective Benefits

Curcumin offers various mechanisms for heart protection:[36]
- ✓ It can help lower blood pressure.[37]
- ✓ Curcumin can reverse age-related decline in blood vessel function, thus decreasing the risk of heart disease.[38]
- ✓ Turmeric has been shown to reduce the clotting tendency of blood platelets,[39] as excessive platelet clumping increases the risk of heart attacks.
- ✓ Curcumin enhances heart-related beneficial blood chemicals such as HDL cholesterol and apolipoprotein A while also reducing harmful ones, such as triglycerides, LDL cholesterol, total cholesterol, apolipoprotein B and lipoprotein A.[40]
- ✓ It can be beneficial for patients with heart failure.[41] A common misconception is that heart failure means one's heart has stopped functioning completely. In reality, it

refers to the heart's inability to adequately pump and disseminate blood throughout the body. So heart failure means reduced heart functioning, not complete stoppage.

Anti-Diabetic Benefits[42]

- ✓ Turmeric may reduce blood glucose levels in diabetics.[43]
- ✓ In individuals on the verge of developing diabetes (pre-diabetics), turmeric has been shown to prevent progression to full-blown diabetes.
- ✓ Turmeric improves pancreatic function and counters insulin resistance.[44]
- ✓ Curcumin may help stave off diabetic cataracts, which can form in the eye lens of diabetics.[45]
- ✓ Curcumin may prevent diabetes-induced medical complications.[46] Long-term high blood glucose levels can cause damage when glucose reacts with body proteins to form advanced glycation end products (AGEs). This can result in retinal damage, kidney and nerve damage, heart disease, fragile bones (osteoporosis), rheumatoid arthritis and accelerated ageing.[47]
- ✓ Turmeric may help slow the progression of kidney damage caused by diabetes, known as diabetic nephropathy.[48]
- ✓ Recent research suggests that consuming turmeric along with different diabetes medicines can improve blood glucose levels and reduce nerve damage.[49]

Digestive Health Benefits[50]

- ✓ For thousands of years, turmeric has been used to enhance digestion, relieve gas and eliminate worms.
- ✓ It prevents stomach ulcers.[51] Turmeric contains compounds that protect the stomach mucus lining and kill a strain of bacteria that causes stomach ulcers. Oxidative

stress and this bacterial infection reduce mucus secretion and increase stomach acid, leading to stomach ulcers. Although there are medications to treat this condition, they can have side effects.[52]
- ✓ Turmeric boosts immunity by promoting the growth of beneficial bacteria in the intestines.
- ✓ Curcumin has been found to reduce the relapse rate in patients with an intestinal disorder called ulcerative colitis.[53]
- ✓ Irritable bowel syndrome, characterized by abdominal pain, diarrhoea or constipation, has been linked to stress, anxiety and a previous intestinal infection. Turmeric can help alleviate its symptoms.[54]

Immunity Benefits

Turmeric possesses antibacterial, antifungal, antiviral and anti-parasitic properties.[55]

Joint-Protective Benefits

- ✓ Turmeric can help with osteoarthritis – an inflammatory joint condition – thanks to its anti-inflammatory compounds.[56]
- ✓ Curcumin has been shown to be more effective than diclofenac sodium, a common NSAID painkiller, in treating rheumatoid arthritis without side effects.[57]

Respiratory Benefits

Turmeric's anti-inflammatory compounds can improve some inflammatory respiratory conditions, such as allergic asthma and chronic lung diseases like chronic obstructive pulmonary disease (COPD).[58]

Reproductive System Benefits

Taking 200 mg of curcumin daily for ten days can significantly reduce the severity of premenstrual syndrome's emotional, behavioural and physical symptoms.[59]

HOW TO CONSUME

Turmeric can be incorporated into curries and soups and be used for frying or pickling. It can also be added to both sweet and spicy dishes.

Fresh Turmeric Root

This yellow root, similar to ginger but smaller, is widely available. After washing and scraping off the peel, the core can be chopped into small pieces or grated. But most people prefer to use turmeric in its powdered form for convenience.

Turmeric Powder

The dried root can be ground into a fine, dark-yellow turmeric powder, which is ideal for seasoning curries and other dishes. While it's easily available in stores, some people prefer to purchase dry turmeric roots and grind them at home.

Turmeric Tea

To make turmeric tea, add a quarter teaspoon (about 1 g) of turmeric powder to a cup of boiling water and simmer for 3 minutes. To enhance the flavour, add honey or fresh lemon juice.

Turmeric Milk

Turmeric lattes are gaining popularity around the world, but Ayurveda has long recommended drinking turmeric milk before bedtime. Simply combine half a teaspoon turmeric and half a teaspoon ghee or clarified butter, then stir into warmed milk.

Turmeric Supplements

This is the most reliable method of using turmeric for medicinal purposes, and the reasoning behind it will be discussed later in this chapter.

HOW TO SELECT

- ✓ Fresh turmeric roots look like ginger but are slightly smaller in size.
- ✓ Choose firm roots or rhizomes and avoid any that are soft or shrivelled.

Turmeric Powder Adulteration

Unfortunately, turmeric powder is often adulterated. It is frequently combined with fillers such as chalk powder, sawdust, rice powder or starch to increase volume. Bright synthetic colours, such as metanil yellow, lead chromate, acid orange or Sudan red, are occasionally used to enhance the powder's vibrant yellow hue. Sometimes, raw or wild turmeric is mixed in.[60] These additives render turmeric hazardous and unfit for consumption.

Identifying contamination solely by sight can be difficult. But here are some relatively simple tests you can conduct at home:[61]

- ✓ **Palm test:** Rub a pinch of turmeric powder on your palm for fifteen seconds. Turn your palm upside down. If pure, the turmeric will stick and leave a yellow stain. If most of the powder falls, it could be adulterated.
- ✓ **Water test:** Mix a teaspoon of turmeric powder in a glass of warm water. If the powder settles to the bottom after fifteen minutes and the water remains pale yellow, it is most likely genuine. If the powder does not settle and the water turns a darker yellow, it could be adulterated.
- ✓ **Turmeric root test:** To test a turmeric rhizome (not the powder), place it on paper and sprinkle with water. If it is artificially coloured, some of the colour may leach onto the paper.[62]
- ✓ **Lead chromate test:** Dissolve a teaspoon of turmeric in water. Lead chromate, being water soluble, will instantly impart a yellow tint to the water.

For those willing to wear a scientist's hat and perform slightly more complex tests, you can try these:

- ✓ **Starch test:** Under a microscope, genuine turmeric particles are large and yellow with sharp edges, whereas starch particles are small, white and round.
- ✓ **Metanil yellow test:** Mix a teaspoon of turmeric with hydrochloric acid and gently shake. If the mixture contains metanil yellow, it will turn pink.
- ✓ **Chalk powder test:** If a turmeric and hydrochloric acid mixture produces bubbles, it indicates the presence of chalk powder.

To avoid adulterated turmeric, buy turmeric roots and grind them at home as needed. If this is impractical, choose a reputable turmeric powder brand. Avoid buying loose turmeric powder.

HOW TO STORE

- ✓ Fresh turmeric can be stored in an airtight container in the refrigerator for up to two weeks.
- ✓ To store for several months, place it in the freezer inside a plastic bag.

HOW MUCH TO CONSUME[63]

- ✓ Curcumin accounts for approximately 4 per cent of turmeric by weight. One teaspoon of turmeric, weighing about 3 g, contains approximately 120 mg of curcumin.
- ✓ To enhance curcumin absorption, eat turmeric with fat-rich meals.
- ✓ For optimal results, consume curcumin in three equal servings per day. Curcumin has a half-life of 6–7 hours in our blood, so it is eliminated from the body shortly after consumption. Dividing doses helps maintain stable blood curcumin levels.
- ✓ A daily intake of **500 mg** of curcumin is recommended for overall health. This translates to around 12 g (4 tsp) of turmeric a day. In contrast, a typical Indian diet contains 2 to 3 g (1 tsp) of turmeric.
- ✓ Consuming 12 g turmeric daily may not be convenient. Furthermore, it is unclear if consuming 12 g per day for a long period is safe. Therefore, we recommend **6 g (2 tsp)** of turmeric per day.

✓ For medicinal benefits, higher doses are required. Typically, **1,500 mg** of curcumin per day is advised, which comes to about 36 g (12 tsp) of turmeric daily, a massive quantity. Since consuming more than 6 g of turmeric a day is not recommended, we will discuss an alternate solution below.

A Case for Turmeric Supplements

Consuming 12 to 36 g of turmeric daily is not possible through diet alone. Furthermore, curcumin has a very low (less than 2 per cent) absorption rate in the intestine.[65] No wonder then that turmeric is one of the most under-appreciated medicinal foods in the world.

However, there are simple, modern solutions. Turmeric or curcumin supplements can be an effective alternative because they usually contain 100 per cent curcumin extract – roughly twenty-five times more potent than the powdered form. Just 1.5 g of curcumin extract would be sufficient for daily medicinal use.

Various proprietary technologies can significantly improve curcumin bioavailability (intestinal absorption).[66] For example, mixing it with piperine, a compound found in black pepper, can boost the absorption of curcumin from 2 to 40 per cent.[67]

In other words, a **75 mg** curcumin supplement blended with piperine provides the body with same amount of curcumin as **1.5 g** of unblended curcumin extract or 36 g (12 tsp) of turmeric powder per day.

Thus, if you want to reap the full medicinal benefits of turmeric, curcumin supplements are your best bet.

HOW MUCH IS TOO MUCH

- ✓ The US Food and Drug Administration (FDA) classifies turmeric and curcumin as GRAS (Generally Recognized As Safe).
- ✓ Even at doses as high as 12,000 mg daily, unblended curcumin does not produce harmful side effects.[68] However, it is best to avoid more than **8,000 mg** of curcumin extract a day.
- ✓ If you opt for blended curcumin, adjust this number for the increased absorption ratio. For example, do not exceed **200 mg** of curcumin blended with piperine.
- ✓ When it comes to turmeric, do not consume more than **12 g** a day to prevent side effects.

WHO SHOULD AVOID

- ✓ Turmeric contains high quantities of oxalates, which, when combined with calcium, can form some types of kidney stones.[69] Curcumin supplements, however, can help avoid this problem as they do not contain oxalate compounds.
- ✓ Individuals with iron deficiency problems should limit turmeric intake as its oxalates can bind with iron, reducing its absorption.
- ✓ Curcumin stimulates the gallbladder to release more bile and empty out,[70] helping prevent gallstones. However, those with gallstone blockages in the bile duct may experience intensified pain due to this effect.
- ✓ Those who take blood-thinning medicines should restrict their consumption of turmeric as it inhibits clotting.

- ✓ Individuals undergoing elective surgery should reduce turmeric consumption two weeks before and after the procedure to avoid the risk of excess bleeding.
- ✓ High turmeric intake can negatively affect foetal growth in pregnant women.[71] It can also cause menstrual cramps and stimulate uterine contractions, leading to premature delivery or miscarriage.
- ✓ Breastfeeding women should not consume excess turmeric since its effects on infants are unknown.
- ✓ The structure of curcumin is similar to the female hormone oestrogen, mimicking it in the body. Patients of hormone-sensitive cancers such as breast, uterus and ovaries, or conditions like uterine fibroids or endometriosis, should limit their turmeric consumption since the common treatment for such conditions is reducing blood oestrogen levels.
- ✓ On the other hand, if you are on oral contraceptives or undergoing oestrogen replacement therapy, in which the aim is to raise blood oestrogen levels, you should still limit turmeric consumption as it may also show anti-oestrogenic properties – for a more in-depth explanation, refer to the flaxseeds chapter.
- ✓ Excessive curcumin can reduce blood glucose levels, which, combined with diabetes medicines, can lead to hypoglycaemia.
- ✓ Taking large amounts of turmeric can cause stomach upsets, nausea and diarrhoea. Prolonged intake may even lead to stomach ulcers.[72]
- ✓ While turmeric improves sperm quality in men, overconsumption might lower testosterone levels, impairing sperm mobility and overall male fertility.[73]
- ✓ High consumption of turmeric can cause liver damage.[74]

SUMMARY

Systems and Benefits	Major	Minor
Anti-inflammatory	■	
Antioxidant	■	
Bones		
Brain	■	
Cancer	■	
Diabetes		■
Digestive	■	
Eyes		
Heart	■	
Immunity	■	
Joints		■
Liver	■	
Mental Health		■
Pregnancy & Lactation		
Reproductive		■
Respiratory		■
Skin & Hair	■	

Consumption:

- Use **6 g** (**2 tsp**) turmeric through foods daily.
- For medicinal use, **1,500 mg** of ordinary (unblended) curcumin per day, divided over three equal doses.

Excess: Avoid more than **12 g** turmeric a day.

10

CARROT
Eye Specialist

In the late 1500s, the northern Dutch Low Countries, reeling under Spanish control, erupted in revolution. And William of the House of Orange-Nassau emerged as the powerful leader of the rebels.

Following an eighty-year-long struggle, the Dutch Republic eventually became an independent country. To honour William's contributions, orange was adopted as the national colour of the Netherlands.

Around this time, the Dutch were an agricultural powerhouse in Europe. To assert their brand, some Dutch farmers decided to flood the European markets with orange-coloured produce from their country, aiming to subliminally assert, 'Think orange, think Dutch'.

Unfortunately, hardly any local vegetables were naturally orange, until one farmer noticed a curious mutation: orange carrots, previously unseen.

The commonly consumed carrots in those days were purple. But they had two drawbacks: they stained hands and cookware and turned brown when cooked. The Dutch farmers wondered:

could they cultivate this orange variety locally? Would it satisfy European palates? They were eager to experiment.

The results surpassed expectations. Not only did orange carrots grow well in the mild, wet Dutch weather, they tasted delicious without leaving any stains. Soon, the Netherlands was exporting orange carrots by carriage loads. Thanks to their innovation, even today, the most common colour of carrots remains orange. Maybe we, too, should 'think carrots, think Dutch'.

Carrot (*Daucus carota*) is a vegetable prized for its edible taproot. It belongs to the plant family of cumin, dill and parsnips, all characterized by their umbrella-like flower clusters. The origins of carrot can be traced to Persia – modern-day Iran – where it used to be cultivated for its stems and leaves. The earliest varieties had small, tough and woody taproots, which, after centuries of selective breeding, have grown larger, less fibrous and tasty. Now, they come in various shapes – from elongated to bulbous – and their tips are blunt or pointed. They can be eaten raw or cooked – each method offering its own advantage, as discussed later in the chapter.

NUTRIENTS

Carrots have 88 per cent water, 9.6 per cent carbohydrates, 0.9 per cent proteins and 0.2 per cent fats.[1]

Nutrition in Suggested Daily Amount of **Carrot**		Eat **100** grams
		Has **41** calories
Source	*Nutrient*	*Daily Need (%)*
Great	*Vitamin A equivalent*	83.5
	Vitamin K	24.0
Good	*Vitamin B$_9$ (folate)*	9.5
	Vitamin C	7.4
	Manganese	7.2
	Dietary Fibres	7.0
	Vitamin B$_6$ (pyridoxine)	6.9
	Potassium	6.8
	Vitamin E	6.8
	Phosphorous	5.8
	Vitamin B$_3$ (niacin)	5.5
	Vitamin B$_5$ (pantothenic acid)	5.5
Poor	*Vitamin B$_1$ (thiamine)*	4.7
	Sodium	4.6
	Magnesium	4.0
	Vitamin B$_2$ (riboflavin)	3.6
	Calcium	3.3
	Copper, zinc, iron and selenium	Less than 3

Carrots are available in purple, yellow, red and orange colours. Each type is loaded with a different plant nutrient:

- ✓ Purple carrots are rich in anthocyanins, which are cancer-preventive antioxidants.
- ✓ Yellow carrots are packed with lutein and zeaxanthin, eye-protective antioxidants.

- ✓ Red carrots are rich in lycopene, a heart-protective antioxidant.
- ✓ Orange carrots are full of carotenes, nutrients that convert into vitamin A in our body. Carotenes serve as great antioxidants that reduce oxidative stress and degenerative damage. Therefore, they offer protection against heart disease, brain degenerative disease, some cancers and age-related eye damage.

While our school textbooks state that carrots are a great source of vitamin A, they don't actually contain vitamin A, a significant advantage that will be discussed later in this chapter.

HEALTH BENEFITS

Carrots possess antioxidant, anti-inflammatory, anti-cancer and anti-diabetes properties. They are beneficial for the eyes, skin, heart, bones, immunity and reproductive system.[2]

Antioxidant Benefits

Many internal body processes and external sources, such as pollution, UV rays and cigarette smoke, can alter our cell DNAs. These changes can cause degenerative damages, accelerate ageing and trigger heart disease, cancer and brain disorder.

Carotenes, lutein, lycopene and anthocyanins – antioxidants found in different varieties of carrots – are highly effective against oxidative damage.[3] Therefore, carrots are likely to be beneficial in many degenerative conditions.

Eye-Protective Benefits

Every kid learns that carrots are good for the eyes. Before talking about these benefits in detail, though, let's first see what carrots can't do for your vision:

Myopia (Nearsightedness)

Contrary to popular belief, eating carrots cannot get rid of your eyeglasses! Myopia is caused by elongation of the eyeball – a mechanical issue that cannot be solved nutritionally by carrots or any other food. Barring this misconception, however, carrots offer various other benefits for other aspects of eye health.[4]

Night Blindness

- ✓ The vitamin A in carrots helps create a light-sensitive protein critical for vision in low light. The first symptom of vitamin A deficiency is often difficulty seeing in low light. This deficiency, if untreated, can lead to night blindness.
- ✓ Low levels of this protein can delay how quickly your eyes adjust to low light. For a person experiencing a vitamin A deficiency, shifting from a brightly lit area to a darker one can be challenging. Eating carrots regularly can readily mitigate this problem.

Colour Blindness

Vitamin A helps form another protein needed for colour perception, so its deficiency can also lead to colour blindness – a condition remedied by consumption of carrots.

Cataracts

Cataracts occur when the lens of the eye becomes cloudy, affecting sight. Its onset is usually age-related.
- ✓ Vitamin A can help reduce the risk of developing age-related cataracts.[5]
- ✓ Their progression can be slowed through daily intake of carotenes with other nutrients.[6]

Age-Related Macular Degeneration (AMD)

High blood concentrations of carotenes may aid in preventing AMD, a condition where the retina gets damaged, causing loss of vision.[7] Both lutein and zeaxanthin, found only in orange and yellow varieties of carrots, are known to protect against AMD.

Glaucoma

It's noteworthy that eating carrots twice a week can decrease the chances of developing glaucoma by 64 per cent![8]

As explained earlier in the book, glaucoma can lead to progressive loss of vision or blindness. But this is a mechanical issue, not a nutritional one. So how do carrots help with it?[9]
- ✓ One possibility is that people eating carrots tend to be health-conscious and may exercise more, which helps reduce pressure inside the eyes.
- ✓ Another factor is the presence of lutein. As discussed in the chapter on spinach, lutein helps in managing glaucoma.[10] When oxidative stress blocks the fluid drainage vents in the eye, pressure builds up inside the eye, causing glaucoma. As an antioxidant, lutein can prevent or control this problem.[11]

Dry Eyes

In cases of dry eyes disorder, the eyes cannot produce enough tears to stay adequately lubricated. The tears may be of poor quality, and the tear film itself may be unstable. This can cause eyes to become dry, develop redness, burning, itching and light sensitivity.

Carrots contain vitamin A, which can aid in managing dry eyes:
- ✓ Lack of vitamin A can lead to dry, wrinkled eye surface, potentially causing eye ulcers and even blindness.
- ✓ Vitamin A can help treat dry eyes by promoting the formation of an eye-lubricating tear film.[12]

Skin-Protective Benefits

The skin cells act as the body's first defence against external threats such as pathogens, toxins and even sunlight. Similar protective cells guard the inner linings of our lungs and intestines, and the exterior surfaces of all organs, blood vessels and internal cavities. Another set of barricades are the mucous layers inside the nose, sinuses, mouth, inner ears, lungs, intestines, urinary tract, bladder and vagina.

Carrots and vitamin A maintain the health of body barriers like the skin, organ linings and mucus layers.[13]

Recent research shows how exactly vitamin A benefits the skin. For practical reasons, though, these studies used readymade vitamin A, rather than carrots. Since the amount of vitamin A used in the trial was similar to that found in carrots, it is possible that the latter will also provide these benefits.

Better Skin

- Carrots contain vitamin A, which promotes the growth of new blood vessels in the skin,[14] improving nutrient supply and skin tone.
- They stimulate the production of proteins that make the skin firm (collagen) and elastic (elastin), protecting it against acne and wrinkles.[15]
- They aid in removing old, damaged skin protein fibres.

Dry Skin

Deficiency of vitamin A causes the skin to become dry, itchy and scaly, increasing the risk of cracks and infections.

Wounded Skin

- Vitamin A can partially repair damaged skin by rebuilding its structure, making it more resistant to cuts, bruises, and sunburns.[16]
- It also aids in various stages of wound healing.[17]

Abnormal Growth of Skin Cells

Conditions involving abnormal growth of skin cells can benefit from vitamin A, as it can help manage the outermost layer of the skin, with the tough structural protein keratin and dead skin cells that are constantly being shed. New cells form at the base of this layer and as the cells above them are shed slowly, they move to the surface over four to eight weeks before starting to shed themselves.

In certain conditions, skin cells may produce excess keratin, causing the topmost layer to thicken. This can often lead to blistering or rough skin, as seen in cases of psoriasis.

Psoriasis

Vitamin A can regulate keratin production, which decreases the formation of abnormal skin patches.[18] It also reduces the toxic chemicals that cause inflammation in psoriasis.

Acne

Vitamin A can alleviate common teenage issues like facial acne. Its deficiency results in excessive keratin production at hair roots, blocking the removal of dead skin cells and skin oil. This can lead to acne. Vitamin A helps clear debris and oil from the skin pores, preventing acne and reducing subsequent scarring.

Skin Cancer

Vitamin A lowers the risk of a common type of skin cancer. Of course, skin cancer is more prevalent in countries with predominantly white-skinned populations. Within the Indian subcontinent, our brown skin acts as a natural protective shield.[19]

Protection of Mucous Membranes

- ✓ Vitamin A helps maintain healthy mucous membranes. Its absence may cause those surfaces to lose their protective properties.[20]
- ✓ Deficiency of vitamin A can dry out the urinary tract and vaginal lining, causing burning sensations and bleeding, which is a common issue in women after menopause.[21]
- ✓ This deficiency can make people more susceptible to respiratory infections.[22] It occurs when the lining of the lungs and windpipe (trachea) loses its protective function.
- ✓ By protecting these linings, vitamin A also reduces the harmful effects of air pollution.[22]

Digestive Benefits

Dietary fibre improves digestive health, while also benefitting the body's immunity and nervous systems. A hundred grams of chopped carrots provide nearly 7 per cent of your daily fibre requirement!

Weight-Loss Benefits

Carrots are high in dietary fibre, which means that eating them keeps you fuller for longer periods. Furthermore, they are low in calories, but since this is true for many other bland foods, this is a comparatively insignificant benefit.

Heart-Protective Benefits

- ✓ Eating carrots may lower the risk of heart disease, as the vitamins B_6 and B_9 present in carrots can reduce homocysteine, a blood chemical linked to increased heart disease risk.[23]
- ✓ Consuming carotenes from fruits and vegetables may lower the blood levels of inflammatory chemicals like c-reactive protein (CRP).[24] Chronic and excess inflammation is a recognized cause of heart disease.
- ✓ The dietary fibre in carrots reduces cholesterol absorption in the intestines, helping control blood cholesterol.
- ✓ Carrots may reduce the risk of plaque formation, a process in which fats, cholesterol and other substances accumulate in the walls of the blood vessels and narrow the arteries, restricting blood flow. Lower levels of plaque in arteries have been linked with high carotenoid levels in the blood.[25]

- ✓ They are a good source of potassium, which counteracts the adverse effects of sodium on heart function and relaxes blood vessels, lowering blood pressure.

Anti-Diabetes Benefits

- ✓ The fibres in carrots slow down glucose absorption in the intestines, resulting in better blood glucose control in diabetes.[26]
- ✓ By reducing blood glucose absorption, keeping you from overeating and aiding weight loss, carrots can help prevent and control diabetes.
- ✓ Vitamin A deficiency increases the risk of developing diabetes.[27]
- ✓ Long-standing diabetes can lead to complications such as diabetic neuropathy, where high blood glucose levels cause nerve damage, leading to pain and numbness, digestion problems, loss of bladder control and irregular heart rates. Being high in many B-vitamins, carrots are believed to aid nerve health.
- ✓ People with type 2 diabetes are often found to have low levels of vitamin B_6,[28] which carrots provide in good measure.

Immunity-Protective Benefits

The vitamin A content in carrots plays a significant role in our immunity.[29]
- ✓ It stimulates the production of new white blood cells, which serve as the body's army in resisting infections.
- ✓ Vitamin A regulates the body's immune response,[30] which prevents food allergies from being triggered.

✓ Carrots contain vitamin C, which helps boost our immunity.[31]

Anti-Cancer Benefits

Carrots have many plant compounds that have been proven to protect against certain cancers.
✓ Carotene-rich diets protect against prostate,[32] colon,[33] breast[34] and stomach[35] cancers.
✓ Vitamin A reduces the risk of cervical,[36] breast,[37] pancreatic,[38] bladder[39] and lung[40] cancers.[41]
✓ Purple carrots contain anthocyanins that have many proven cancer-preventive properties.[42] Currently, the challenge is their poor absorption in the body.
✓ Red and orange carrots have lycopene, which has been extensively studied for its role in cancer prevention and control.[43]

Since cancers are life-threatening diseases, medical science needs far more robust proof of carrots' efficacy against them than, say, for healthy skin. So, this benefit is still under considerable research.

Note: Please don't alter your cancer treatment without discussing it with your doctor.

Reproductive System Benefits

Vitamin A is necessary for the proper development of a human foetus's heart, lungs, kidneys, eyes, pancreas and nervous system. But both an excess or deficiency of vitamin A can be harmful. Irregularities in the concentration of vitamin A in a mother's body can lead to birth defects, potentially causing physical deformities and mental retardation.

> **Why Should Pregnant Women not Drink Alcohol?**
>
> Even though it is unusual for a pregnant woman in India to consume alcohol, it's important to understand why it should be avoided. The liver converts alcohol into a chemical bearing similar properties to vitamin A. This chemical circulates in the bloodstream for a few hours after alcohol consumption and may be mistakenly taken up by body cells looking for vitamin A. In pregnant women, the tissues of the developing foetus can make this error, resulting in the uptake of the alcohol by-product, which is useless, instead of the required vitamin A. The foetus can then suffer consequences similar to those caused by a vitamin A deficiency, potentially leading to birth defects, as a growing foetus cannot tolerate such shortfalls as effectively as an adult body.

- ✓ Vitamin A supports the male genital tract and proper sperm production.[44]
- ✓ A vitamin A deficiency can detrimentally affect the female reproductive system by lowering egg quality. In such cases, the egg may also fail to implant in the uterus, potentially leading to a miscarriage.[45]

✓ Vitamin A supports human reproduction and is required at almost every stage of the embryo development, underscoring its vital role in pregnancy.[46]

Why did we not discuss the vitamin A benefits in the earlier chapter on spinach, another substantial source of vitamin A? Considering their typical daily consumption, carrots provide 84 per cent of the daily requirement of vitamin A, while spinach just offers 35 per cent.

Bone-Protective Benefits

When discussing bone health, calcium and vitamin D usually come to mind. But vitamin A? Who has even heard of it in relation to bone health before? New research suggests that vitamin A keeps our bones healthy in two ways:
1. Vitamin A helps produce collagen, a protein that provides structure, support and strength to the bones.
2. As an antioxidant, vitamin A has the potential to slow the degenerative process that weakens bones.

It's important not to consume vitamin A in excess, as evidence suggests that both a deficiency and an overabundance of vitamin A can increase the risk of bone fractures. In other words, your bones are at their healthiest when you consume the right amount of vitamin A each day – neither too much nor too little.[47] Overdosing on vitamin A can surely break (pun unintended!) the party.[48]

This is where carrots can come in handy. Carotenes are believed to reduce the risk of bone fractures. But they do it more effectively than vitamin A – even if you eat too many carrots by mistake, you won't increase the risk of bone fractures. The underlying reason for it is explained later in this chapter. So, for better quality bones, increase your carrot intake.

HOW TO CONSUME

- ✓ The green leaves of the carrots, while edible, are rarely consumed.
- ✓ While you can choose to drink carrot juice, it's better to avoid it as the juicing process removes fibre, which has health benefits.
- ✓ Carrots can be eaten raw, peeled, chopped or grated. They can be sautéed for biryanis, minced for fillings, sliced for soups and stews, shredded for frying or roasted and served with meats.
- ✓ Given their mildly sweet taste, carrots find their way into desserts like cakes and puddings. Most famously, they're used to prepare *gajar ka halwa*, a staple North Indian dessert with a simple recipe.[49] But it would be improper for a health-oriented book to discuss high-sugar carrot desserts further!
- ✓ Onions, shallots, garlic, cucumbers, chives, apples, beets and meats go well with carrot. It can also be seasoned with herbs such as coriander, parsley and cilantro.[50]

Should You Cook Carrots?

The answer depends on various factors. Cooking destroys at least one-third of the vitamin C in carrots, but it's unlikely that you consume carrots purely for their vitamin C content.

Carotenoids such as lutein and zeaxanthin are bound rigidly within the carrot fibres. For the body to absorb them, they need to be released. If carrots are consumed either raw and crunchy or lightly steamed, most of their carotenoids cannot be absorbed in the intestines.[51]

One study suggests that the absorption of carotenes is only 3 per cent from raw carrots, 21 per cent when the carrots are pulped, 27 per cent when the pulp is cooked and 39 per cent when the cooked pulp is mixed with cooking oil.[52]

When it comes to food, let us not focus on the exact numbers. Every carrot variety is distinct due to differences in harvesting methods and so on. Plus, every meal is different, given the diversity in preparation methods and accompanying foods. The key takeaway is that cooked carrots provide more carotenoids than raw ones.

So don't be a bunny rabbit; cook your carrots!

HOW TO SELECT

- ✓ A quality carrot has firm, plump skin with a deep, consistent colour.
- ✓ Avoid any that are rubbery or display signs of over ripeness, such as cracks, soft spots or small strings at the

- bottom (rootlets), as these carrots are past their prime.[53]
- If the leaves are still attached to the carrots, make sure they're fresh, bright and lively. Wilted leaves mean the carrot has been sitting on the shelf for too long.
- Regular carrots are both sweeter and healthier than baby carrots.

HOW TO STORE

- Cut off the green leafy tops, as carrots lose moisture through them.
- Keep them in unsealed plastic bags in the refrigerator to prevent from rotting. This way, they will last two weeks.
- Don't store them near bananas and apples as the latter two produce gases that can overripen carrots.
- To deep-freeze, chop them into smaller cubes before storing. These pieces can last eight to nine months.
- Refrigerating them uncooked can cause them to lose nutrients, colour and flavour over time. Therefore, before storing them, blanch the carrots in the following way:[54]
  1. Wash and peel them. Then cut them into thin slices, long strips or small cubes. Leave the smaller carrots whole.
  2. Simmer them in boiling water for two minutes.
  3. Cool them quickly in ice-cold water before draining, packing, sealing and freezing.[55]

Given that carrots are widely available all year, blanching may be worthwhile only if you plan on carrying them on an Antarctic expedition, though!

HOW MUCH TO CONSUME

There are no established recommendations for consuming carrots or carotenes. However, there are guidelines for vitamin A intake. In the US, men and women are advised to consume 900 and 700 μg of vitamin A daily, respectively.[56] In India, the recommended values are a little higher: 1,000 μg for men and 840 μg for women.[57]

A 100 g carrot contains approximately 830 μg of vitamin A. But isn't this confusing, given that we previously stated that carrots, like most plant foods, do not contain vitamin A? So, where does this vitamin A come from?

As mentioned earlier, carrots contain carotenes, which the body uses to produce vitamin A. In nutritional science, the convention is to refer to the total vitamin A body gets as a result, instead of the carotene quantity. This vitamin A is expressed as retinol activity equivalents (RAE), with retinol being a form of vitamin A. Thus, it's more accurate to say that 100 g of carrots contain about 830 μg RAE of carotenes.

This is why the nutritional tables at the beginning of every chapter list 'Vitamin A equivalent', not 'Vitamin A'.

Despite the fact that carrots are high in vitamin A, many other foods are rich in it. As a result, it is recommended that you limit your carrot consumption to about **100 g** daily. It's also okay to skip carrots three to four times per week.

A Case for Carotene Supplements

Carotenes in plant foods are fat-soluble, which means they are better absorbed when combined with fats. So, carrot-rich meals must include at least a few grams of fat.

On the other hand, supplemental carotenes are extracted from plants and combined with healthy oils, enhancing their absorption by almost sixfold. To put this into perspective, 100 g of carrots contain 10,000 µg beta-carotene, which provides 830 µg of vitamin A to your body. A supplement containing just 1,667 µg beta-carotene provides comparable vitamin A levels.[58] Common beta-carotene supplements contain 6,000 µg beta-carotene. Thus, it is much easier to meet your vitamin A requirements with a beta-carotene supplement than with carrots, especially when you are travelling, sick or simply dislike eating carrots.

Furthermore, if the supplements contain significantly higher quantities of carotenes than your daily requirement, it will not cause toxicity, as explained in the next section.

HOW MUCH IS TOO MUCH

To avoid toxicity, consume no more than **3,000 µg** of vitamin A per day.[59]

You can get vitamin A indirectly from carrots and carotenes (called provitamin A) or directly as vitamin A (preformed vitamin A) through animal sources such as organ meats and cheese. Consuming too much vitamin A can lead to a condition called hypervitaminosis A, which can cause irreversible damage.[60]

On the other hand, when you consume carotenes, your body converts only what it needs into vitamin A. This way, you never hit the toxic upper limit of vitamin A, regardless of how much carotenes you consume.[61]

Think of it like buying rice: it is better to get uncooked rice and prepare only as much as you need, instead of risking excess by purchasing it cooked.

Of course, this doesn't mean you should eat lots of carrots every day. Overconsumption of beta-carotenes can result in carotenemia, a condition where the skin turns orange.

Avoid eating more than **200 g** of carrots per day, though even this amount will not turn your skin orange. If you eat ten medium carrots (400 g) a day for two weeks, orange carotenes may get deposited in areas with thicker skin, such as your palms, elbows and nasal folds.[62] It is most noticeable in people with lighter skin tones. But luckily, it is fully reversible by stopping any consumption of carotenes.

WHO SHOULD AVOID

- ✓ People allergic to carrots, as they may experience swelling or difficulty in breathing. (If you are reading this book, you probably know if you have such an allergy.)
- ✓ While carrots are safe for children as a food, large amounts of carrot juice may not be safe for young children, especially infants.
- ✓ Breastfeeding women may eat carrots but should avoid carrot juice for the same reason.
- ✓ Since carrots are high in dietary fibres, a rapid increase in carrot intake may result in constipation, bloating and abdominal pain.

SUMMARY

Systems and Benefits	Major	Minor
Anti-inflammatory		■
Antioxidant	■	
Bones		■
Brain		
Cancer		■
Diabetes		■
Digestive		■
Eyes	■	
Heart		■
Immunity		■
Joints		
Liver		
Pregnancy & Lactation		■
Reproductive		■
Respiratory		
Skin & Hair	■	

Consumption: **1** large carrot (**100 g**) two to three times a week.

Excess: Don't consume more than **2** large carrots (**200 g**) daily.

11

FLAXSEEDS
Omega-3 Powerhouse

Textile production is a massive global industry today. But when did humans learn to make fabric? Since all kinds of fibres disintegrate over a few thousand years, it is difficult to identify their original materials. Until recently, the oldest evidence was fabric impressions in clay, carbon-dated to be around 25,000 years old, but there was no way to know which material they were made of.

In 2009, however, a critical discovery was made by scientists while excavating soil samples in Dzudzuana Cave in Georgia. They found over a thousand fibres of flax that had been preserved thanks to the humid air inside the cave in the foothills of the Caucasus mountains. Carbon-dating would reveal them to be over 30,000 years old.

Some of the fibres were twisted, indicating they had been spun and woven. Other were dyed black, grey, turquoise and even pink, suggesting an astounding degree of craftsmanship.

It is plausible that our hunter-gatherer ancestors used these fibres to stitch animal hides into warm clothing and shoes. They may have also tied objects together with ropes made of fibres, so that they could carry more items or create nets for hunting.

Thus, flax gave us the world's oldest known textiles. They probably also increased the survival chances of our forefathers almost 36,000 years ago.[1]

Flaxseeds come from the flax or linseed plant (scientific name *Linum usitatissimum*). This versatile plant has dual uses. It can be cultivated as a food source or woven into linen, a fabric two to three times stronger than cotton. When used to make clothes, paints or ink, it is referred to as linseed; as a dietary item, it is called flaxseed. The plant was first seen in Mesopotamia (modern-day Iraq) around 5,000 BCE and, since then, it has been grown and used in many parts of the world.

NUTRIENTS

Flaxseeds are 7 per cent water, 29 per cent carbohydrates, 18 per cent proteins and 42 per cent fats.[2]

Nutrition in Suggested Daily Amount of **Flaxseeds**		Eat **15 grams**
		Has **80 calories**
Source	*Nutrient*	*Daily Need (%)*
Good	*Magnesium*	19.6
	Manganese	18.6
	Vitamin B_1 (thiamine)	17.6
	Phosphorous	16.1
	Dietary Fibres	10.2
	Selenium	9.5
	Copper	9.2
	Vitamin B_9 (folate)	6.5

	Zinc	3.8
	Calcium	3.8
	Vitamin B_6 (pyridoxine)	3.5
	Iron	3.0
Poor	*Vitamin B_5 (pantothenic acid)*	3.0
	Potassium, vitamin B_3 (niacin), vitamin B_2 (riboflavin), vitamin K, vitamin E, sodium, vitamin C and vitamin A equivalent	Less than 3

Besides vitamins, minerals and dietary fibres, flaxseeds also contain:

- ✓ **Alpha-Linolenic Acid (ALA):** An essential omega-3 oil, which protects the heart and exhibits anti-inflammatory and anti-diabetes properties. ALA is helpful against kidney disease, ulcerative colitis, rheumatoid arthritis, migraine headaches, depression, eczema, psoriasis and respiratory conditions such as pneumonia and chronic obstructive pulmonary disease (COPD).[3] Nearly half of the fats, 22 per cent of flaxseeds, are ALA. Fifteen grams of the seeds contain 3.4 g of ALA, more than double our daily requirement. Since excess ALA is not harmful, flaxseeds serve as a safe and excellent source.
- ✓ **Proteins:** Most vegetarian foods are not very high in protein, with flaxseeds being the exception. Nearly one-fifth of their weight comprises high-quality proteins,[4] on a par with soybean protein.[5] Since flaxseeds are gluten-free, they are suitable for people sensitive to gluten. If you eat the daily recommended amount of 2 tbsp of flaxseeds, you will only get about 3 g of proteins. This isn't enough to meet your daily protein needs, which are between 40

and 80 g. But you can consume flaxseed flour, with fat removed (de-fatted), to obtain this benefit.[6]
- ✓ **Lignans:** Show antioxidant, anti-inflammatory, anti-cancer, anti-menopausal and heart-protective benefits.[7] Flaxseeds contain 75 to 800 times more lignan than other plant foods.[8]

    Lignans are different from lignins – the former are plant compounds digested in the intestines, while the latter are indigestible compounds found in all types of wood.[9]

Flaxseed oil is extracted from flaxseeds after removing their fibres and proteins. Two tablespoons (15 g) of flaxseeds yield 1/2 tbsp (7 ml) of flaxseed oil.

HEALTH BENEFITS

Traditional Benefits

Flaxseeds and their oil have been used in Ayurveda for millennia.

Flaxseeds:

- ✓ They balance skin pH, increase skin elasticity and hydration, heal blemishes and wounds and treat skin problems like dryness, premature wrinkles and dullness.[10]
- ✓ They are known to boost overall health, immunity and brain function while improving physical endurance, muscle strength and vitality by alleviating fatigue and controlling aging.
- ✓ According to Ayurveda, flaxseeds can help treat disorders caused by the imbalance of vata dosha in the body, like nerve pain, paralysis, constipation and bloating.[11]

Flaxseed Oil:

- ✓ It can improve strength and immunity.
- ✓ When applied externally, the oil detoxifies the skin.
- ✓ Flaxseed oil has uses in enema, as a massage oil or as ear and nasal drops.
- ✓ Like the seeds, flaxseed oil can also be used to treat diseases caused by the imbalance of vata dosha.

Modern Benefits

New research indicates that flaxseed oil, as well as its fibres and lignans, can help in combatting heart disease, diabetes, breast and colon cancers, arthritis, fragile bones (osteoporosis), along with some neurological and immunity-related disorders.[12]

Anti-Inflammatory Benefits

ALA and lignans in flaxseeds can inhibit the release of certain inflammation-causing chemicals. This could help with various conditions that are linked to inflammation, such as plaque buildup, asthma and Parkinson's disease.

Heart-Protective Benefits

- ✓ Regular consumption of flaxseeds can lower systolic and diastolic blood pressures.[13] This is because they contain ALA and certain plant proteins.
- ✓ Eating flaxseeds regularly may reduce total and LDL cholesterol and raise the HDL levels.[14] This benefit is due to the presence of ALA, flax fibres and lignans. Notably, flaxseed oil, lacking fibres and lignans, offers only marginal benefits in this regard compared to the seeds.

- ✓ The antioxidant properties of flaxseed lignans (rather ALA) prevent the oxidation of LDL cholesterol. Flaxseed oil cannot provide this benefit as it does not have any lignans.
- ✓ ALA can reduce inflammation in the blood vessels, making them more resistant to developing heart disease.
- ✓ Flaxseeds inhibit the ability of platelet cells to stick to each other.[15] This reduces the clotting tendency of the blood.
- ✓ These benefits work together to reduce plaque formation inside blood vessels (atherosclerosis). Flax lignans are believed to reduce plaque buildup by up to 75 per cent.[16]
- ✓ Flaxseed may help treat irregular heartbeats (arrhythmia) and heart failure as ALA has shown potential to normalize heartbeat. But further research is needed to confirm this benefit.

Please seek proper medical care for heart failure or arrhythmia. You should not try treating these conditions on your own.

Anti-Cancer Benefits

- ✓ Flaxseeds appear to protect against cancers of the breast,[17] colon,[18] blood,[19] lungs[20] and prostate[21].
- ✓ The ALA in flaxseeds may prevent tumour formation and growth.[22]
- ✓ Flax lignans lower the risk of developing hormone-dependent cancers, such as breast cancer, from a young age.[23] They block the female hormone oestrogen, reducing its biological activity and harmful effects in young women before menopause.

- ✓ Lignans also help reduce the risk of non-hormone-dependent cancers, like colorectal cancer.[24] This is due to their antioxidant and anti-inflammatory properties.[25]
- ✓ Additionally, lignans protect against the spread of tumour cells (metastasis) because of their antioxidant properties.[26]

Digestive Benefits

Fifteen grams of flaxseeds contain 4 g of dietary fibre, which is 10 per cent of your daily need. This makes them a good source of dietary fibre.

- ✓ Insoluble flax fibres help bulk up the food in the intestines, improve bowel movements and ease constipation. They also stimulate the relaxation and contraction of intestinal muscles (peristalsis).[27]
- ✓ Soluble fibres can absorb excess water in your gut and swell. If cases of loose motions, soluble fibres help solidify the intestinal mass, thereby controlling the diarrhoeal symptoms.[28]
- ✓ Flaxseeds have a 70:30 ratio of insoluble to soluble fibres. So, they help alleviate both kinds of problems: insoluble fibres for constipation and soluble for diarrhoea.[29]
- ✓ ALA and lignans can help ease the symptoms of irritable bowel syndrome. These benefits can be obtained from the seeds but not from flaxseed oil as it lacks fibres and lignans.

Many other benefits of dietary fibres are covered in detail in the chapter on sabja (sweet basil) seeds.

Anti-Diabetes Benefits

- Flaxseed intake has been found to reduce blood glucose,[30] primarily by lowering glucose absorption in the intestines.
- It also decreases insulin resistance.[31]

Weight-Loss Benefits

The high fibre content in flaxseeds slows the stomach emptying rate without reducing satiety.[32] According to one study, people who consumed 30 g – double the recommended daily amount – of flaxseeds, experienced significant reductions in their body weight and waist measurement.[33] However, consuming this much may cause digestive discomfort.

Bone-Protective Benefits

- Consuming flaxseeds can improve bone health.[34]
- Some researchers found that flaxseeds may even be more effective than the combination of calcium and vitamin D.[35] Why is this the case?

New studies indicate that the health of our bones depends on many factors besides calcium deposition. Bones are living tissues, with the calcium within their structures being continuously removed and redeployed by specific bone cells. When diets are high in inflammatory foods (processed foods, simple carbohydrates and sugars, vegetable oils and trans fats), calcium removal from bones is higher, thus weakening them. In contrast, consuming more anti-inflammatory foods can strengthen the bones by preventing their deterioration.[36]

The anti-inflammatory properties of ALA prevent bone breakdown or resorption. Ongoing trials are trying to quantify this benefit.[37]

HOW TO CONSUME

Flaxseeds can be eaten whole, crushed or ground as a powder (with fat) or flour (without fat), while flaxseed oil can be consumed as a liquid or a supplement capsule.[38]

HOW TO SELECT

- ✓ Flaxseeds are available in two varieties, brown and golden. Both offer similar flavours and benefits,[39] with the brown variety being more widely available, and having a crunchier, stronger taste. Golden flaxseeds are comparatively lighter, creamier and sweeter.
- ✓ When buying readymade flaxseed flour or powder, choose products in an opaque packaging with distant expiry dates. This is because the ground powder, also known as milled flaxseed or flax meal, can turn rancid within weeks of opening the packet.
- ✓ Buy flaxseed oil only in dark-coloured bottles as it can spoil quickly when exposed to sunlight. Unless you plan to consume significant quantities, opt for smaller bottles. Ensure that the expiry date on the packaging allows you to finish the oil before it.

HOW TO STORE

- ✓ Store whole flaxseeds in a cool, dark place for up to a year. Refrigeration is the most effective method for extending their shelf life.
- ✓ To keep flaxseed flour or powder fresh for several months, store it in an airtight container in the refrigerator.[53] It can even be kept inside the deep freezer.

- ✓ If you prefer to buy whole flaxseeds and grind them yourself, do it right before use. The freshly ground powder should be refrigerated in an airtight container.
- ✓ Flaxseed oil should ideally be stored in a bottle inside the fridge to maintain freshness.

HOW MUCH TO CONSUME

- ✓ It's generally recommended to consume **2 tbsp** (**15 g**) of flaxseeds per day.
- ✓ Many medical studies have used 4 to 5 tbsp of ground flaxseed powder. However, for most people, 2 tbsp per day over a long period should suffice.
- ✓ Some people prefer to eat flaxseeds whole, without chewing them. But this way, they pass through the body undigested. As our bodies are unable to break down whole seeds, you won't receive any nutritional benefits. Instead, chew the seeds thoroughly or grind them into a powder before swallowing them.
- ✓ A simple home coffee or spice grinder can be used to make flaxseed powder. But since the ground form spoils faster, mill the seeds right before use.
- ✓ Ingest flaxseeds with water, as they can cause constipation otherwise.
- ✓ Alternatively, ½ **tbsp** (**7 ml**) of flaxseed oil can be consumed every day. Although this provides an equivalent amount of ALA (3.4 g), the oil lacks the proteins, fibres and beneficial lignan compounds found in the seeds. So, if given a choice, choose flaxseeds over oil.
- ✓ Consuming rancid flaxseeds or flaxseed oil can potentially cause inflammation and cholesterol-related issues.

- ✓ Avoid heating flaxseed oil while cooking, as it has a very low smoking point (107°C or 225°F). Heating beyond this point can cause the oil to burn and its compounds to degrade.[40] Add the oil to your dish only after the food has finished cooking. Also, don't reheat such dishes in the microwave afterwards.

HOW MUCH IS TOO MUCH

- ✓ Do not exceed a daily intake of more than **5 tbsp (40 g)** of flaxseeds per day.
- ✓ Do not consume more than **2 tbsp (30 ml)** of flaxseed oil in a day.
- ✓ Flaxseeds and flaxseed oil are safe and generally have no side effects when consumed in their recommended amounts.
- ✓ Overconsumption of flaxseeds can lead to gastrointestinal discomfort, such as gas trouble, bloating, cramping and loose motions.
- ✓ Flaxseeds contain trace amounts of cyanides and cadmium, which are typically harmless in such quantities. But to avoid health risks associated with their buildup, do not eat too many flaxseeds per day.[41]

WHO SHOULD AVOID

- ✓ Individuals with breast, ovarian and uterine cancers should avoid flaxseeds due to their mild oestrogenic effects, which may promote cancer growth.[42] This is because the lignans present in flaxseeds act as phytoestrogens, meaning the plant compounds start to mimic oestrogen. Medical treatments for these cancers prevent the body from producing oestrogen or stop the hormone from binding to the body cells by blocking their hormone receptors.[43] Consuming flaxseeds and their lignans might prove detrimental in such a situation. Conversely, some new evidence suggests that phytoestrogens can protect against these cancers.[44] With the science still evolving, it is wiser for those suffering from any of these cancers to avoid eating flaxseeds.

- ✓ Flaxseed oil does not have any phytoestrogens and poses no risk in the cases of hormone-sensitive cancers.
- ✓ On the other hand, in some cases, flaxseeds demonstrate anti-oestrogenic effects. If you are on oral contraceptives or are undergoing oestrogen replacement therapy, where the aim is to raise oestrogen levels, you should limit the consumption of flaxseeds.[45] If you still want to include them in your diet, wait an hour or two after taking the medicine or therapy session.

Are Flaxseeds Oestrogenic or Anti-oestrogenic

We've discussed above the dual effect of flaxseeds: oestrogen-like on certain cancers and anti-oestrogen-like on contraceptive medicines. But how can they possess both traits?

Flaxseed compounds behave like oestrogen when the body is facing its shortage and compete with oestrogen when it is in abundance.

Our body cells feature oestrogen receptors, where the hormone typically binds, initiating its effects. During cancer treatments that lower natural oestrogen levels, many receptors are left unoccupied by oestrogen, creating an opportunity for flaxseed compounds to bind and trigger an oestrogen-like response.

However, when there is sufficient oestrogen in the body, the flaxseed compounds compete with it to latch on to the same receptors. Since flaxseed lignans are mildly oestrogenic, every cell receptor with a phytoestrogen attached to it in lieu of regular oestrogen causes diminished oestrogen action, effectively acting as an anti-oestrogenic.

Think of oestrogen like a professional and phytoestrogens like amateurs. At a disaster site, prior to the arrival of the rescue team, the bystanders aid in relief work. But once the professionals reach, the same helpers may become a hindrance to the recovery efforts.

✓ Avoid flaxseeds during pregnancy or breastfeeding as:
 1. In the second or third trimester of pregnancy, they may increase the risk of premature birth.[46]
 2. There is limited information about the safety of flaxseeds for infants who are breastfeeding.
 3. The safety of consuming flaxseeds and flaxseed oil during pregnancy remains uncertain. Some websites and experts claim they are safe, others say they are not. National Institutes of Health (NIH), USA, suggests that they may be unsafe due to their mild oestrogenic effects.[47] American College of Obstetricians and Gynecologists (ACOG), on the other hand, states that flaxseeds and flaxseed oil are good sources of omega-3

oils in pregnancy, implying their consumption is fine.[48] Adding to the complexity, some government authorities advise not to exceed 1 tbsp of flaxseeds a day and to avoid flaxseed oil altogether.[49] Our view, yet again: when in doubt, stay out.

- ✓ Flaxseeds can reduce blood clotting, so it is best to avoid them at least two weeks before and after elective surgeries.
- ✓ Individuals on blood-thinning medicines should be careful.
- ✓ Individuals on blood glucose-lowering medicines should eat flaxseeds cautiously, as they can amplify the effects of these drugs, potentially causing hypoglycaemia.
- ✓ Be careful when using flaxseed oil if you're also taking antihypertensive medicines, as their combination can reduce blood pressure excessively.
- ✓ Flaxseeds can interfere with the absorption of many oral medicines, so remember to consume them at least two hours apart from taking any medicine.
- ✓ People allergic to flaxseeds should refrain from both the seeds and the oil, as intake could result in reactions like itching, redness, shortness of breath, nausea and vomiting.

SUMMARY

Systems and Benefits	Major	Minor
Anti-inflammatory	■	
Antioxidant		■
Bones		■
Brain		■
Cancer	■	
Diabetes		
Digestive		■
Eyes		
Heart	■	
Immunity		■
Joints		■
Liver		
Mental Health		
Pregnancy & Lactation		
Reproductive		
Respiratory		
Skin & Hair		■

Consumption: 2 tbsp (15 g) of flaxseeds or **½ tbsp (7 ml)** of flaxseed oil a day.

Excess: 5 tbsp (40 g) of flaxseeds or **2 tbsp (30 ml)** of flaxseed oil daily.

12

AMLA
(INDIAN GOOSEBERRY)
Immunity Superstar

Sri Adi Shankara, a revered Indian philosopher, was born in the small town of Kaladi (in the south Indian state of Kerala) in the eighth century. As a boy of eight, he adopted the practice of sannyas (renunciation) and bhiksha (begging for alms, an act of subduing one's ego).

One day, while seeking alms, he stood in front of the hut of a poor woman. The lady searched her entire house but found nothing to offer except an amla. She did not want to send away the hermit empty-handed, so she placed the fruit in his begging bowl.

Struck by her selflessness, Sri Adi Shankara started singing hymns in praise of Goddess Lakshmi. The legend goes that the goddess, pleased by his devotion, showered the poor woman's home with amla fruits made of gold.

These twenty-one stanzas of praise are called the 'Kanakdhara Stotram'. 'Kanak' means gold, 'dhara' signifies flow and 'stotram' is a eulogy. It is believed that regularly chanting this paean can bring about great fortune.[1]

Even 1,200 years later, that house remains standing in Kalady, underlining how amla has figured in Indian history, folklore and mythology for millennia.

Amla, also known as Indian gooseberry, is a fruit borne by a flowering tree (scientific name *Phyllanthus emblica*). This tiny, round and translucent yellow-green fruit is known for its distinctive flavour – a combination of sour, bitter and astringent, with a sweet aftertaste.

Amla's natural habitat extends across the Indian subcontinent, from Myanmar in the east to Afghanistan in the west, and from the northern foothills of the Himalaya to the Deccan plateau in the south.

NUTRIENTS

Each Amla fruit weighs between 60 and 70 g. It is composed of 86 per cent water, 10 per cent carbohydrates, 1 per cent proteins and 0.5 per cent fats.[2]

Nutrition in Suggested Daily Amount of **Amla Fruits**		Eat **100 grams**
		Has **48 calories**
Source	*Nutrient*	*Daily Need (%)*
Great	Vitamin C	598
	Dietary Fibres	12.5
	Vitamin A equivalent	9.7
Good	Vitamin B_5 (pantothenic acid)	6.0
	Vitamin B_6 (pyridoxine)	5.0
	Copper	5.0
	Manganese	5.0

	Potassium	4.2
	Phosphorous	3.5
	Magnesium	3.3
	Iron	3.1
Poor	*Vitamin B_9 (folate)*	3.0
	Calcium, Vitamin B_1 (thiamine), Vitamin E, Selenium, Vitamin B_3 (niacin), Sodium, Zinc, Vitamin B_2 (riboflavin) and Vitamin K	Less than 3

Amla is a rich source of vitamin C, a water-soluble vitamin. Any excess consumption is excreted in the urine, causing no long-term harm.

The other potent plant compounds in amla are:

- ✓ **Quercetin:**[3] Contains antioxidant,[4] anti-inflammatory,[5] anti-allergic,[6] anti-cancer,[7] brain-protective[8] and heart protective properties[9]
- ✓ **Kaempferol:** Antioxidant, anti-inflammatory, anti-cancer and antimicrobial effects. It is known to protect the heart, brain, bones, liver, lungs and digestive system.[10]
- ✓ **Gallic acid:** Antioxidant, anti-inflammatory, anti-cancer, anti-obesity and anti-microbial benefits.[11] It also helps with digestive, heart and brain disorders.[12]
- ✓ **Ellagic acid:** Antioxidant, anti-inflammatory, anti-cancer and anti-diabetes properties. It is also known to protect the brain, heart, skin and improve immunity.[13]

HEALTH BENEFITS

Traditional Medicinal Uses

Amla has been a staple in Ayurveda, known as *divyaushada* or divine medicine, for millennia. According to Ayurveda, the three humours or doshas in our body must be balanced in order to treat a variety of diseases.[14] A common ingredient in many *rasayanas*, or rejuvenating tonics, amla is one of the three fruits that can help achieve this balance.

Ayurvedic experts have long extolled the virtues of amla for addressing the following conditions:[15]

- ✓ Digestive system disorders: constipation, haemorrhoids, heartburn, gastritis, colitis, colic and dyspepsia
- ✓ Metabolic disorders: diabetes, gout, anaemia
- ✓ Lung disorders: asthma, cough
- ✓ Bleeding disorders: blood in the urine, bleeding gums, ulcerative colitis, heavy and prolonged menstrual bleeding
- ✓ Ageing disorders: fragile bones, weak vision, premature grey hair
- ✓ Inflammation, fever, burning sensations
- ✓ Physical and mental exhaustion, fatigue, palpitations, mental disorders, vertigo

We will focus on the modern-research-based benefits of amla. But we must acknowledge the wisdom amassed over centuries. In fact, a lot of traditionally known benefits can be explained by a current understanding of the composition of amla.

Modern Medicinal Uses

Antioxidant Benefits

Amla contains many antioxidant compounds that protect the body from free radical damage.[16] It helps avoid or delay degenerative disorders such as heart disease, diabetes and cancer, and improves immunity. These conditions are partially interlinked – what protects a person from one will also protect him from the others.[17]

Anti-inflammatory Benefits

✓ Amla has excellent anti-inflammatory properties that are effective against both chronic and acute inflammation.[18] This is thought to be due to its phenolic compounds like gallic acid.[19]
✓ Many pharmaceutical painkillers work by lowering inflammation. But one of their side effects is that they also damage the digestive tract,[20] which is why scientists are still researching natural anti-inflammatory agents. Foods such as amla, with few side effects, show promise in this quest.

Immunity-Related Benefits

✓ The vitamin C in amla can improve immunity,[21] warding off various infections.[22]
✓ Gallic acid, ellagic acid and kaempferol can also help boost immunity.

Digestive Benefits

✓ Amla is rich in pectin, a water-soluble dietary fibre that promotes bowel movements.[23]
✓ It can alleviate the severity of symptoms linked with digestive conditions like irritable bowel syndrome.

- ✓ Vitamin C improves the absorption of iron and selenium, which means consuming amla may benefit this process. But do not overindulge as excessive vitamin C can also impede the absorption of copper, nickel and manganese.[24]
- ✓ Amla has anti-diarrhoeal properties, potentially helping with stomach cramps.[25]
- ✓ Contrary to the belief that amla exacerbates acidity (heartburn) due to its sourness, research indicates that it can actually reduce the frequency and severity of acidity in individuals who already suffer from stomach acid-related issues.[26]
- ✓ It may even help prevent stomach ulcers[27] or heal them.[28]

Anti-Cancer Benefits

- ✓ Amla boasts of more than a dozen compounds with cancer-protective properties.[29]
- ✓ It can increase the activity of protective immune cells against various types of tumours.[30]
- ✓ The ellagic acid in amla can prevent DNA damages, the leading trigger for cancers.[31]
- ✓ Amla prevents the growth and spread of breast, uterus, pancreas, stomach and liver cancers.[32]
- ✓ It may also alleviate the side effects of cancer treatments such as chemotherapy and radiation therapy.[33]

Please note that amla is not a treatment for cancer but can be considered for preventive or supportive use. It's essential to consult your doctor before incorporating it into your daily routine if you are undergoing cancer treatment.

Liver-Protective Benefits

Early stages of fatty liver involve fat accumulation in the liver, a condition called non-alcoholic fatty liver disease (NAFLD). If left uncontrolled for a couple of years, liver can develop inflammation causing non-alcoholic steatohepatitis (NASH). And if unchecked for two to four more years, it can even result in severe liver damage and eventually cirrhosis. Fatty liver is often linked to people with obesity.

- ✓ Amla may help prevent the onset of fatty liver and related conditions.[34]
- ✓ Inflammation and oxidative stress can cause liver damage. Since amla can protect the body against both, it can also prevent liver injury.[35]

Anti-Diabetes Benefits

- ✓ Amla contains pectin, a fibre that slows down glucose absorption in the intestines after a meal, reducing post-meal blood glucose spikes.
- ✓ Research suggests that amla can lower blood glucose levels as well as lipids (cholesterol and triglycerides) in patients of diabetes.[36]
- ✓ Antioxidant compounds in amla can safeguard against the onset of diabetic complications, resulting from prolonged high blood glucose levels, that affect the heart, kidneys, eyes and nerves.[37]
- ✓ In cases of diabetes, elevated blood glucose levels can lead to eye cataracts. However, the tannins in amla can help protect against diabetic cataracts.[38]
- ✓ High blood glucose levels can damage the inner lining of blood vessels in people with diabetes, even resulting in

heart disease. Amla promotes vascular health by reducing inflammation and preventing damage to the blood vessels.[39]

Heart-Protective Benefits

- ✓ Amla helps lower blood pressure.[40]
- ✓ Thanks to its water-soluble pectin fibre content, amla reduces cholesterol absorption in the intestines.
- ✓ It may also lower the levels of blood cholesterol and other fats.[41]
- ✓ Amla reduces the presence of inflammatory chemicals associated with a higher risk of heart disease.
- ✓ It decreases the blood's clotting tendency.[42]
- ✓ Amla can potentially protect the heart through various other mechanisms.[43]

Brain-Protective Benefits

- ✓ It may enhance learning and memory.[44]
- ✓ Amla might improve brain function in people with memory loss[45] – its vitamin C content boosts the production of a brain chemical called norepinephrine, which is found to prevent or delay the development of dementia.[46]
- ✓ It can reduce free radical activity in the brain,[47] possibly preventing conditions like Alzheimer's disease.

Kidney-Protective Benefits

- ✓ Amla may protect against age-related kidney damage.[48]
- ✓ It might also safeguard against kidney damage caused by various toxins and free radicals.[49]

Hair-Protective Benefits

- ✓ Amla can reduce hair loss and increase growth[50] by inhibiting a chemical called 5-alpha reductase that causes male and female pattern baldness.[51]
- ✓ It stimulates the production of specific hair cells that support hair growth.[52]
- ✓ The deficiencies of iron, selenium and vitamins B_9 and B_{12} have been linked to premature greying or whitening of hair.[53] Since amla is rich in many of these nutrients, it may help prevent greying as well.

Skin-Protective Benefits

- ✓ The antioxidants present in amla can shield the skin from free radical and oxidative damage, reducing the appearance of fine lines and wrinkles.[54]
- ✓ These antioxidants contribute to healthier and more robust skin.[55]
- ✓ The vitamin C found in amla supports various other aspects of skin health as well.[56]

Eye-Protective Benefits

- ✓ Amla may help protect against cataracts,[57] which are accelerated by free radicals, neutralizing them through the antioxidant properties of vitamin C and tannins.
- ✓ It may protect against cellular damage associated with age-related macular degeneration – a condition that impairs retinal cells and leads to vision loss.[58]
- ✓ Amla can also be used as a home remedy for treating conjunctivitis or 'pink eye', an inflammatory condition of the eyelid.[59] This is due to its inflammation-reducing vitamin C and bioflavonoid contents.

Please do not apply amla juice directly to the eyes, though, as it can cause severe damage. The above benefits can be realized by regularly consuming the fruit or its juice.

Various claims also suggest that amla can improve reproductive and mental health, as well as prevent pain and aid in weight loss. But there is almost no modern scientific evidence to support these claims and, thus, we will not delve on them.

HOW TO CONSUME

Amla can be enjoyed fresh, dried, preserved, pickled or candied. It's also available as dried powder or juice. Harvested between October and February, amla is a seasonal fruit.[60]

- ✓ **Amla preserve** is made by cooking fully matured whole fruits in sugar syrup until they become transparent and tender.[61]
- ✓ **Amla jam** is prepared by extracting pulp from the fruit, then mixing it with sugar and citric acid before cooking it to a thick consistency.
- ✓ Amla can be mixed with salt and sun-dried over several days. Commercially, it can also be oven-dried with hot air. The **dried whole fruit** can then be turned to flakes, slices, shreds or powder.
- ✓ **Amla juice**, known for being pungent due to its high vitamin C content, is often mixed with other fruit juices like grapes, apples, lime, ginger or pomegranate for better palatability.
- ✓ **Amla candies** extend the fruit's storage life while retaining its nutritional value. The process involves dipping the fruit in a salt solution, washing and blanching, steeping

in sugar syrup, coating with sugar and drying in the shade thereafter.
- ✓ **Amla sauce** can be made from amla pulp combined with tomato pulp, sugar, salt, onions, garlic, ginger, red chillies and hot spices.
- ✓ Small amla fruits that are unsuitable for preserves and candies can be used for making **amla pickles**.[62] The fruits are brined to reduce their astringent taste and admixed with oils and spices before being left to dry in the sun for a few days.

Alternatively, amlas can also be baked into tarts, and its juice can be used to flavour vinegar and marinades.[63]

HOW TO SELECT

- ✓ Choose ripe amla fruits that have a slightly firm, yellowish-green skin.
- ✓ Look for ones that are round with vertical stripes.
- ✓ Avoid selecting any with black or brown spots, bruises, cuts or patches on the skin.

HOW TO STORE

- ✓ If kept outside, the fruit can last for about five to six days.[64]
- ✓ Stored in the refrigerator, it should remain fresh for around two weeks.
- ✓ Jams, squashes and jellies made from amla can easily last up to nine months.[65]
- ✓ Amla pickle can be stored at room temperature.

HOW MUCH TO CONSUME

- No specific dosage applies to amla and its variants, but experts generally recommend consuming **one** to **two** amla fruits (equivalent to around **100 g**) daily.
- Alternatively, consume **1½ tsp** (**6 g**) of amla powder or **2 tbsp** (**30 ml**) of amla juice daily.
- Preferably split the intake into two equal doses per day.
- Opinions are divided on whether drinking amla juice should be avoided at night. Some experts claim it can cause acidity (heartburn) and disturbed sleep.[66] Others affirm that drinking it at night before sleeping is beneficial.[67] I would suggest that it is best not to consume anything at least two to three hours before sleeping.

HOW MUCH IS TOO MUCH

Overconsumption can lead to dehydration, diarrhoea or an upset stomach. Since no scientific studies suggest a safe cut-off, it's best to avoid eating more than **two** amla fruits, **2 tsp** (**8 g**) amla powder or **3 tbsp** (**45 ml**) amla juice in a day.

WHO SHOULD AVOID

- Consuming amla can reduce BP below safe levels, posing a concern for those with low blood pressure.
- Diabetics should carefully monitor their amla intake since it may enhance the blood glucose-lowering effect of their medicines, leading to hypoglycaemia.
- Due to its blood-thinning properties, those taking anti-clotting medication should be cautious when consuming amla.

- ✓ Those preparing for elective surgeries should stop amla consumption two weeks before and after the surgery to avoid any possibility of excessive bleeding.
- ✓ Individuals experiencing coughing issues should avoid consuming amla.
- ✓ Pregnant or breastfeeding women should also avoid amla consumption as there is insufficient evidence regarding its safety (good or bad). While some nutritionists claim amla is safe during pregnancy, it is always better to err on the side of caution.

SUMMARY

Systems and Benefits	Major	Minor
Anti-inflammatory	■	
Antioxidant	■	
Bones		
Brain		■
Cancer	■	
Diabetes	■	
Digestive	■	
Eyes		■
Heart	■	
Immunity	■	
Joints		
Liver		■
Mental Health		
Pregnancy & Lactation		
Reproductive		
Respiratory		
Skin & Hair	■	

Consumption: On an empty stomach, **one** to **two** fruits (**100 g**), **1½ tsp** (**6 g**) powder or **2 tbsp** (**30 ml**) of juice daily. Divide into two equal doses.

Excess: Avoid more than **two** fruits, **2 tsp** (**8 g**) powder or **3 tbsp** (**45 ml**) juice in a day.

13

PINEAPPLE
Joint-Protective Sentinel

Three centuries ago, pineapples were a status symbol equivalent to today's Instagram-friendly exotic car rentals.[1] Soon after Christopher Columbus brought them from Guadeloupe in the Caribbean to Spain, the fruit became highly sought after all across Europe.

However, due to the tropical climate required for pineapples to thrive, they had to endure a lengthy trans-Atlantic journey to reach Europe, often resulting in spoilage. The solution was the construction of custom-designed hothouses known as pineries, allowing for pineapple cultivation on European soil. Yet, maintaining these pineries to replicate tropical conditions was costly, making these locally grown pineapples more expensive than their Caribbean counterparts. Prices skyrocketed, reaching an estimated £10,000 or 10 lakh per fruit (in today's currency)![2]

Soon, even the rich deemed eating such a precious commodity wasteful. Since pineapples do not ripen if harvested raw, the upper classes took to using raw pineapples as centrepieces at their dinner parties, discarding them once they began to rot.

Then some enterprising individuals hit upon a brilliant idea: pineapple rentals. Commoners, who wanted a part of this spiny luxury, could lease a pineapple for display at events and return it afterwards to the lender. Not too different from today's designer bag rentals!

Eventually, with the advent of steamships to import pineapples from the colonies to Europe, their prices crashed. Now, pineapples are a common sight in fruit markets around the world.

But even today, a giant pineapple dome adorns the main entrance of the National Gallery in London's Trafalgar Square – a monument to mankind's eternal need for status symbols.[3]

Pineapple is a tropical plant (scientific name *Ananas comosus*) that originated in the Brazilian rainforests. For centuries, it has been cultivated in South America and used in folk medicine to treat indigestion and reduce inflammation. In the Caribbean, pineapples are regarded as symbols of friendship and hospitality.[4] Across Asian cuisine, its culinary use is extensive, often featuring in meat, fish, rice and vegetable dishes.

NUTRIENTS

Pineapple Fruit

Pineapple fruit has 86 per cent water, 13 per cent carbohydrates, 0.5 per cent proteins and 0.1 per cent fats.[5] The water content varies from 83 to 92 per cent depending on the fruit variety. So take these numbers as averages.

Nutrition in Suggested Daily Amount of **Pineapple Fruit**		Eat **165 grams**
		Has **83 calories**
Source	*Nutrient*	*Daily Need (%)*
Great	*Vitamin C*	98.6
	Manganese	76.5
Good	*Vitamin B_9 (folate)*	14.9
	Vitamin B_1 (thiamine)	9.3
	Vitamin B_6 (pyridoxine)	9.2
	Copper	9.1
	Vitamin B_5 (pantothenic acid)	7.0
	Magnesium	6.6
	Dietary Fibres	5.8
Poor	*Vitamin B_3 (niacin)*	4.6
	Potassium	3.8
	Vitamin B_2 (riboflavin)	3.3
	Phosphorous, calcium, vitamin K, iron, zinc, vitamin A equivalent, selenium, vitamin E and sodium	Less than 3

The pineapple fruit has many beneficial plant compounds:

- ✓ **Polyphenols:** Exhibit antioxidant, anti-inflammatory, anti-cancer and anti-diabetes properties. They also protect the heart, brain, bones and digestive system.[6]
- ✓ **Bromelain:** A powerful cocktail of enzymes that are anti-inflammatory, anti-cancer and anti-microbial.[7] Bromelain helps the digestive, cardiovascular and respiratory systems[8] and is particularly effective for joint protection.[9] It also has low toxicity, high efficiency and significant absorption in the intestines (bioavailability). Notably, pineapple is the only edible plant in the world that contains bromelain.

Pineapple Juice

Pineapple juice has 84 per cent water, 16 per cent carbohydrates, 0.5 per cent proteins and 0.1 per cent fats.[10]

Nutrition in Suggested Daily Amount of **Pineapple Juice**		Drink **250** ml
		Has **150** calories
Source	*Nutrient*	*Daily Need (%)*
Great	Manganese	140.0
	Vitamin C	29.7
Good	Vitamin B_1 (thiamine)	17.0
	Magnesium	11.7
	Copper	10.8
	Vitamin B_6 (pyridoxine)	9.3
	Potassium	6.5
	Vitamin B_9 (folate)	6.3
	Vitamin B_5 (pantothenic acid)	5.0
	Dietary Fibres	5.0
Poor	Vitamin B_3 (niacin)	3.9
	Calcium	3.5
	Vitamin B_2 (riboflavin)	3.0
	Phosphorous, selenium, iron, zinc, vitamin K, vitamin A equivalent, vitamin E and sodium	Less than 3

Drinking the juices of foods that are typically eaten whole isn't always ideal, as they contain fewer fibres crucial for our digestive system. However, despite sacrificing some fibre content, consuming more pineapple juice can offer higher quantities of certain nutrients compared to eating the fruit itself.

HEALTH BENEFITS

Pineapples come with a host of health benefits, attributed to their antioxidant, anti-inflammatory, anti-cancer and analgesic properties. They boost immunity, protect joints, aid digestion and maintain heart health.

Anti-Inflammatory Benefits

Pineapples can reduce inflammation due to their bromelain content.[11]

Joint-Protective Benefits

Joint pain is a leading cause of debilitation among older adults, often resulting from weak cartilage. Pineapples can offer significant benefits in preserving healthy joint cartilage.

Joint Cartilage

Cartilage is a strong yet flexible tissue that cushions the ends of bones at joints. It serves as a lubricant when the bones rub against each other, preventing painful friction, as observed in arthritis. Cartilage also acts as a shock absorber, easing the strain of activities like running or jumping on the body.

Unlike inert attachments such as hair or nails, cartilage is a living tissue. Similar to bones and muscles, it strengthens with activity and exercise.[12] Conversely, lack of activity can lead to cartilage thinning.[13]

How Does Cartilage Get Damaged?

Too much pressure on the cartilage can lead to rupture.[14] Even though normal activities strengthen cartilage, improper movement or severe impact on the joint can cause harm. When cartilage gets damaged due to age or accident, inflammatory chemicals are produced within the joint, resulting in swelling.[15] This persistent inflammation accelerates the breakdown of the remaining cartilage.[16]

To heal the joint, the inflammation first needs to be reduced. Trying to restore the cartilage without addressing inflammation is a losing battle, eventually often necessitating a joint replacement surgery.

Bromelain is an exceptional anti-inflammatory compound known for controlling joint inflammation. It helps manage osteoarthritis[17] and rheumatoid arthritis, an autoimmune disease. Both these conditions involve joint cartilage damage and swelling, though for different reasons. Bromelain has been found to:

- ✓ Alleviate knee pain[18]
- ✓ Reduce joint stiffness[19]
- ✓ Mitigate cartilage breakdown and joint inflammation[20]
- ✓ Offer safer alternative to painkillers prescribed for osteoarthritis, with just as much effectiveness[21]

Once inflammation is under control, you can gradually increase your activity level.[22] Evidence suggests that activities like walking, and particularly running, can improve knee cartilage, even if it is already damaged.[23]

In conclusion, joint replacement surgery should be your last option, not the first.

The Real Reason Osteoarthritis Has Become More Prevalent in the World

Graveyards, morgues, skeletons: it might sound like the beginning of a horror film script. In reality, these were essential elements of a scientific study conducted at Harvard University in 2017. Their aim? To solve the mystery behind increased knee degeneration.

At stake was an intriguing question: why has the incidence of osteoarthritis doubled in the last fifty years? The reasons seemed obvious: osteoarthritis is associated with old age, and people live longer in modern times.[24] Plus, obesity has increased by leaps and bounds, which worsens knee arthritis.[25] But the scientists remained unconvinced. They suspected there was more to the story. Their only option was to study obese individuals of the same age who lived centuries ago. Did their knees suffer the same fate as those living with similar levels of obesity today?

Forensic pathologists, putting Sherlock Holmes to shame, can determine if a deceased person had osteoarthritis by looking at their knee bones. With their help, the Harvard researchers compared skeletons from six thousand years ago to recently deceased individuals. This led to a startling discovery:[26] Centuries ago, people with obesity had much lower rates of knee arthritis, suggesting that obesity was not the sole cause of rise in osteoarthritis. So what else was driving this increase?

The researchers looked into modern enemies – the

jogging craze, paved roads, air pollution, processed foods and more – but came up empty-handed. The findings defied all logic: standing for hours, like a traffic policeman, was worse for the knees, while walking and, surprisingly, running were the most beneficial.[27]

Eventually, the answer was narrowed down to an unexpected cause: inactivity![28] With extended hours of desk work, increased reliance on vehicles for transportation and the convenience of household machines, our activity levels have gone down over the last fifty years, escalating the prevalence of osteoarthritis.

These revelations upended the notion that overuse of joints, or 'wear and tear', was the primary cause of knee arthritis. Instead, it appears that reduced movement and insufficient stimulation of our joints are the true offenders.

Digestive Benefits

- ✓ Bromelain breaks down proteins, making them easier to digest and absorb in the intestines.[29] It softens meat by dissolving its collagen fibres,[30] which is why pineapple is often featured in meat dishes.
- ✓ Bromelain is used in some digestive mixes available in the market.
- ✓ Pineapple contains dietary fibre, which promotes digestive health and prevents constipation. It should be consumed with meals for these benefits.
- ✓ Due to its anti-inflammatory properties, bromelain can help reduce intestinal inflammation in diseases like

ulcerative colitis and Crohn's disease,[31] but this requires long-term consumption rather than one-off intake. Pineapple should be consumed on an empty stomach to reap the anti-inflammatory benefits.
✓ Don't devour too many pineapple slices at a time! When you chew them, bromelain breaks down the proteins in the tissues of your mouth, causing the characteristic tingling sensation.

Anti-Cancer Benefits

Cancer is considered a degenerative disease associated with prolonged inflammation and oxidative damage.
✓ Bromelain reduces oxidative stress and inflammation.[32]
✓ Laboratory experiments have shown that bromelain can slow down the growth of cancers of the skin,[33] prostate,[34] colon,[35] breast[36] and the bile duct[37].

But these are early-stage studies, so please do not stop or alter your current medical treatment for cancer. Add bromelain supplements to your regimen only after discussing it with your doctor.

Pain-Killer Benefits

Bromelain is as effective as non-steroidal anti-inflammatory drugs (NSAID) for relieving pain.[38]

Skin-Protective Benefits

✓ Pineapple contains multiple enzymes that can reduce pain and swelling.
✓ Bromelain has been found to repair skin after an injury or surgery, but it requires the application of pineapple flesh on the skin directly. However, in this book, we will focus solely on the health benefits of consuming pineapples.

Immunity-Protective Benefits

✓ Pineapples are packed with vitamin C, a well-known immunity booster.
✓ Bromelain also strengthens immunity.[39]

Heart-Protective Benefits

✓ Vitamin C serves as a good antioxidant, promoting heart health.
✓ Dietary fibres can reduce cholesterol absorption in the intestines.
✓ Bromelain reduces blood-clotting tendencies, thus preventing heart blockages.[40]

Certain sources claim that pineapples can lower blood pressure because of their potassium content, but this is only partially true. A serving of pineapple fruit (about 165 g) offers 180 mg of potassium – accounting for 3.8 per cent of our daily requirement. In contrast, a 250 ml serving of pineapple juice supplies 305 mg of potassium, nearly 6.5 per cent of our needs. The rule of thumb is that anything that gives you less than 5 per cent of your daily needs is not considered a significant source.[41]

Thus, the pineapple fruit is not a good source of potassium, unlike its juice. Similarly, while pineapple juice is beneficial for blood pressure control due to its potassium content, the fruit itself lacks this attribute.

Now, could you eat more pineapple and get more potassium? Sure. Will that aid in blood pressure control? Technically, yes. But there are reasons why suggested daily intakes are established. Exceeding them may confer one additional benefit but cause other problems such as high blood glucose, diarrhoea, abdominal pain or heartburn.

Post-Exercise Recovery Benefits

The body's natural energy production process is inherently inflammatory and releases harmful compounds. When you exercise, your body produces more energy, which causes inflammation and can lead to sore muscles.[42] Consuming pineapple may help in faster recovery from exercise-induced soreness.[43]

Note: Post-workout inflammation stimulates muscles to adapt to the exercise workload. Subduing such inflammation prematurely may result in reduced muscle development.[44] This suggests that eating pineapples to ease post-exercise soreness could be an effective strategy for amateur athletes, but professional athletes should avoid it.

Pineapple

HOW TO CONSUME

- ✓ Never eat unripe pineapples, as they can be poisonous, potentially causing severe diarrhoea and vomiting. Heating them over 70°C (or 158°F) neutralizes their toxic compounds, making unripe pineapple safe to eat when cooked, grilled or microwaved. They can also be used safely for marinating meats before cooking.
- ✓ When using fresh pineapple, start by cutting off the top and base. Then, stand it upright and slice away its skin in downward vertical motions, removing most of it.
- ✓ Inside the flesh, the central cylindrical core is edible, albeit more fibrous and woodier, which is why many prefer to discard it.
- ✓ The pineapple can be juiced or puréed. It can also be grilled, baked or roasted.
- ✓ Pineapple pairs well with meats, seafood, tomatoes, chillies and herbs.[45]

HOW TO SELECT

- ✓ Once harvested, pineapples do not ripen further even if you store them.[46] Do not buy an unripe pineapple unless you want to use it in cooking.
- ✓ The ripe fruit should feel heavy for its size and yield slightly to pressure when gently squeezed. It shouldn't be too hard or soft.
- ✓ The leaves on top should be green and vibrant. Try pulling off a leaf from the centre of the green crown. If it comes out easily, the pineapple is ripe; if not, it is still raw. Use

your discretion – the seller may not like you yanking off leaves from all his pineapples!
- ✓ It should have a pleasant, mildly sweet aroma at the base. A lack of scent may signify an unripe fruit, whereas a sickly sweet smell may indicate an overripe one.
- ✓ A golden-brown colour suggests a ready-to-eat pineapple. But the converse is not true: A ripe pineapple may still have green skin.
- ✓ The eyes of the fruit should be bright, not dark or wrinkled. Avoid fruits with sour or fermented odours, dried leaves, wrinkled skin, cracks, soft spots, leakage or signs of mould.
- ✓ Try to buy a ripe pineapple on the day you want to use it.

HOW TO STORE

- ✓ If stored at warm temperatures, a pineapple will ferment quickly.
- ✓ If stored in the fridge after cutting, it should be consumed within three to four days.
- ✓ In the deep freezer, it can last up to six months.

HOW MUCH TO CONSUME

- ✓ For overall health benefits, consume **one** cup (**165 g**) of pineapple pieces or **one** glass (**250 ml**) of pineapple juice daily.
- ✓ Since bromelain is a blend of various chemicals, its composition and properties vary depending on the part of the pineapple tree from which it is extracted. The quantity and efficacy of bromelain in the fruit is far less than from the core or stem.[47]

- ✓ Enzymes like bromelain are specified in terms of their ability to perform a certain action, not their weight.[48] Bromelain is rated in terms of its digestive strength and the units are gelatin dissolving units (GDU). A standard bromelain extract may have 2,400 GDU/gram. So, 500 mg of such extract will have 1,200 GDUs. If one were to select another extract rated 3,000 GDU/g, they would only need to consume 400 mg to get the same benefit.
- ✓ Consuming bromelain through the pineapple fruit and juice in quantities advised above is sufficient to maintain general health. But for medicinal purposes, eating pineapple fruit or drinking pineapple juice alone will not provide as much bromelain as needed.
- ✓ To improve digestion, take **200–2,000 mg** of bromelain with each meal. Unfortunately, none of the research papers mention the strength of the bromelain extract; only its weight. In absence of that information, we must assume that they are referring to the standard 2,400 GDU/g bromelain extract. Divide the amount equally among all meals.[49]
- ✓ For non-digestive purposes, consume **200–800 mg** of bromelain daily. Distribute it into two to four doses throughout the day and consume on an empty stomach to prevent the proteins from being digested after a meal.
- ✓ If you have joint pain, consume **1,000 mg** of bromelain every day on empty stomach – divided into two doses.
- ✓ It's worth repeating that getting this much bromelain from pineapple fruit or juice is difficult. You should eat pineapple for overall health and consider bromelain supplements for specific therapeutic needs.

HOW MUCH IS TOO MUCH

- ✓ There are no scientific studies on the toxicity of pineapples among humans.
- ✓ But experts advise against excessive consumption, so do not exceed **165 g** of pineapple pieces or **250 ml** of pineapple juice a day.
- ✓ Consuming bromelain up to 12,000 mg/day has not been found to cause any harmful effects.[50] Yet it is better not to exceed **2,000 mg** a day from bromelain supplements.

WHO SHOULD AVOID

- ✓ Bromelain reduces blood-clotting. Consequently, people on blood-thinning medicines should consume pineapples in moderation to avoid the danger of internal bleeding.
- ✓ Avoid pineapples two weeks before and after any elective surgery to prevent the risk of excessive bleeding.
- ✓ Bromelain may also interact with certain antibiotics, seizure medicines (anticonvulsants), anxiety medicines (barbiturates), sedatives (benzodiazepines), insomnia medicines and depression medicines (tricyclic antidepressants). To avoid potential interference, refrain from consuming pineapple at least two hours before and after the scheduled medicine timings.
- ✓ Anyone with diabetes should be cautious about their pineapple intake due to its sugar content. If you are buying pineapple juice, ensure it is unsweetened.

SUMMARY

Systems and Benefits	Major	Minor
Anti-inflammatory	■	
Antioxidant		
Bones		
Brain		
Cancer		■
Diabetes		
Digestive	■	
Eyes		
Heart		■
Immunity		■
Joints	■	
Liver		
Mental Health		
Pregnancy & Lactation		
Reproductive		
Respiratory		
Skin & Hair		■

Consumption: One cup (**165 g**) of pineapple fruit or **one** glass (**250 ml**) of juice daily.

Excess: Don't exceed **165 g** of pineapple fruit or **250 ml** of juice daily. Don't consume more than **2,000 mg** of bromelain a day through supplements.

14

COCONUT
Hair Specialist

The coconut holds a prominent position in Hindu rituals. It is often cracked open before the start of any significant task, an action steeped in symbolism.

It is called shriphal *in Sanskrit, which translates to 'God's fruit'. Considered the sacred symbol of Lord Ganesh, it is also known as* vighnaharta – *the remover of obstacles and guarantor of success in any endeavour.*

At the start of a venture, the husk of a coconut is removed, symbolizing the letting go of materialistic desires. A tuft of fibre is left above the eyes of the coconut, resembling a head with a lock of hair. The coconut is then shattered against a hard surface, signifying the destruction of the ego and an act of humbling oneself before the deity. The opened shell embodies our desire to be reawakened. The flowing coconut water represents all negativity being flushed from one's mind and body. The white flesh of the coconut symbolizes peace and purity.

After offering the broken coconut at the deity's feet, the flesh is distributed among attendees as prasad, a sacred offering.[1] From newly purchased bicycles to spaceships embarking on *lunar missions, the tradition of cracking coconuts has initiated countless Indian journeys, inviting divine blessings.*

Coconut (scientific name *Cocos nucifera*) is the fruit of the coconut tree – a member of the palm tree family. The trees, found in coastal tropical regions, are cultivated for their husk, white kernel, milk and oil. This versatile fruit is also an important ingredient in tropical culinary traditions.

Once its husk is removed, three openings resembling eyes and a mouth on a human face become visible on the coconut's shell. In old Portuguese, this likeness led to the term 'coco', meaning a 'grinning or grimacing face', ultimately birthing the name coconut.[2]

These three openings are from the three carpels – ovule-bearing female reproductive organs of coconut flowers. Two of these openings, known as germination pores, are non-functional and sealed, while the third is soft and operational, allowing a new coconut shoot to emerge from it and contributing to the tree's reproductive cycle.[3]

NUTRIENTS

Fresh Coconut Meat

Fresh coconut contains nearly 47 per cent water, 15 per cent carbohydrates, 3.3 per cent proteins and 34 per cent fats.[4]

Nutrition in Suggested Daily Amount of **Fresh Coconut Meat**		Eat **30 grams**
		Has **106 calories**
Source	*Nutrient*	*Daily Need (%)*
Great	Manganese	22.5
Good	Selenium	7.6
	Dietary Fibres	6.8
	Copper	6.5
	Phosphorous	5.7
	Vitamin B_9 (folate)	3.9
	Magnesium	3.2
Poor	Iron, potassium, zinc, vitamin B_5 (pantothenic acid), vitamin B_1 (Thiamine), vitamin C, vitamin B_3 (niacin), vitamin B_6 (pyridoxine), vitamin E, calcium, sodium, vitamin B_2 (riboflavin), vitamin K and vitamin A equivalent	Less than 3

Controversies Surrounding Fats in Coconut Meat and Oil

Nearly 85 per cent of the calories in fresh coconut arise from its fats, most of which are saturated, leading to two controversies:

1. Do saturated fats cause heart disease?

- ✓ Some medical organizations caution against consuming coconut because their saturated fats increase LDL cholesterol.[5]
- ✓ Recent research papers have cast doubts on this

understanding, claiming that increased levels of LDL cholesterol alone don't necessarily increase the risk of heart disease.[6] Since there is no definitive verdict on this matter, I'll reiterate our old diktat: when in doubt, stay out. If coconut flesh and oil contain saturated fats, do not consume them beyond the recommended amounts.

- ✓ Western dietary guidelines advise keeping saturated fats to less than 10 per cent of daily calorie intake, as it heightens the threat of heart disease.[7] For a typical 2,000-calorie diet, daily saturated fat intake should not surpass 200 calories or 22 g.
- ✓ Consuming 30 g of coconut meat every day will result in 10 g of total fats, out of which 8.5 g are saturated – accounting for 40 per cent of our daily allowance.

This brings us to the second controversy.

2. Are saturated fats (SFs) in coconut different from those in other sources?

Some experts argue that the SFs in coconut vary from those derived from animals.[8] Given that saturated fats are the nutrition world's favourite punch bag, here is a brief primer on the types of SFs and when they are suitable for consumption:[9]

Saturated Fats

They comprise of large molecules with long tails of carbon atom chains – some made of almost twenty-one carbon atoms. Why is this significant? The longer the chain, the more difficult it is for the body to digest them. Digestive enzymes have to break down these molecules into smaller bits before they can be absorbed in the intestines. So, longer-chain saturated fats travel further along the intestines before being adequately broken down. In contrast, shorter chain SFs are absorbed earlier in the intestines.

Herein lies the issue: the early section of the intestines is directly connected to the liver, enabling the absorbed fats to quickly travel to the liver and be used for energy. Fats mopped up in the later parts of the intestines have to take a more circuitous route to the liver, making it difficult for them to be used as fuel. They get stored as fat as a result, contributing to a cycle that can lead to heart disease.

The liver converts shorter-chain SFs into ketones, a healthy energy source offering various health benefits. They aid in weight loss, increase energy and endurance, improve gut health, prevent memory loss and reduce the risk of diabetes.[10] Who would have thought saturated fats could also help lose fat!

Types of SFs

Based on the length of carbon chains, there are three main kinds:
1. **Long-chain saturated fats (LCSF):** 13 to 21 carbons
2. **Medium-chain saturated fats (MCSF):** 6 to 12 carbons
3. **Short-chain saturated fats (SCSF):** less than 6 carbons

To avoid the growing number of acronyms, oils or saturated fats are denoted by 'C', followed by the chain length. For instance, oils labelled as C13 to C21 are considered long-chains and bad for health. C6 to C12 are medium-chain oils – digested quickly and healthier.

What Types of SFs are Found in Coconuts?

Close to half of coconut's fat content is lauric acid (C12),[11] recognized for its antioxidant, anti-inflammatory, antimicrobial and anti-acne properties.[12] Despite being labelled an 'acid', it is essentially a fatty substance.

Is Lauric Acid Healthy?

Lauric acid, categorized as a medium-chain saturated fat, is deemed safe.[13] But is this true?

C12 or lauric acid straddles the border between medium-chain and long-chain SFs. After all, this transition is somewhat arbitrary. Why is C12 healthy and not C13? There's no particular reason. Some studies say that while considered a medium-chain, lauric acid often behaves like a long-chain – and unhealthy – saturated fat.[14]

Since responses from the scientific community on this matter are ambivalent, it's best not to have too much coconut flesh – stick to around **30 g** a day.

A Balanced Way Forward

Here are some important points:
- ✓ Coconut oil raises LDL cholesterol levels.[15]
- ✓ But people living in tropical areas, whose diets consist of various coconut products, do not exhibit an increased risk of cardiovascular disease.[16]

Is it likely that higher levels of LDL cholesterol contribute to heart disease mainly in people consuming modern diets? It seems so.[17]

Think about it: oxidized LDL cholesterol builds up plaque in your arteries if your diet has a lot of processed foods, vegetable oils and trans fats, or if you smoke.[18] Does that sound like a coconut-related issue or a lifestyle one?

The Verdict

Coconut oil is considered safe for heart health, given its historical use and evidence from traditional societies. But in today's world of unhealthy dietary choices, excessive consumption of coconut flesh or oil may pose potential problems.

In other words, those with healthy diets can incorporate coconut into their meals, but if you have unhealthy food and lifestyle habits, try to limit your coconut intake. So, unless you are living in the Tahitian chestnut plantations in French Polynesia, it's advisable to regulate how much coconut you eat!

Dry Coconut Meat

Properly drying fresh coconut meat reduces its water content from 50 to 5 per cent. So, dried coconut meat has roughly double the nutrient content of fresh coconut, as the non-water content of coconut goes from 50 to 95 per cent during the drying process.

Coconut Water

Coconut water differs in nutrient composition compared to coconut flesh: 95 per cent water, 3.7 per cent carbohydrates, 0.7 per cent proteins and 0.2 per cent fats.[19] Consuming it does not raise any concerns regarding saturated fats.

Nutrition in Suggested Daily Amount of **Coconut Water**		Drink **250 ml**
		Has **48 calories**
Source	*Nutrient*	*Daily Need (%)*
Great	*Magnesium*	20.8
	Manganese	17.8
	Sodium	17.5
	Potassium	13.3
	Vitamin B_2 (riboflavin)	8.9
	Phosphorous	8.3
Good	*Vitamin C*	7.5
	Dietary Fibres	6.9
	Selenium	6.3
	Calcium	6.0
	Vitamin B_1 (thiamine)	5.4
	Copper	5.0
	Vitamin B_6 (pyridoxine)	4.0
	Vitamin B_9 (folate)	3.8
Poor	*Iron, vitamin B_5 (pantothenic acid), zinc, vitamin B_3 (niacin), vitamin A equivalent, vitamin E and vitamin K*	Less than 3

Coconut water is packed with vital minerals known as electrolytes, which are crucial for proper muscle function and maintaining hydration. Adding coconut water to your diet can be an excellent way to replenish them. Intense physical activities, like exercise, can lead to excessive sweating, causing a loss of these minerals, muscle cramps (over-contracting) or muscle weakness (under-contracting). Similarly, vomiting or diarrhoea can deplete electrolytes, necessitating restoration.

Coconut water can naturally mitigate such mineral shortfall. But consider the following factors:[20]

- ✓ Excessive sweating during workouts can result in significant sodium loss from the body. While coconut water is sodium-rich, it may not fully replenish the deficit.
- ✓ Drinking copious amounts of coconut water after morning walks is a popular trend. Many people believe that the potassium in it can lower blood pressure. But drinking just two glasses of coconut water can exceed one-third of the daily sodium intake limit, raising the risk of high blood pressure, heart attack and stroke.[21]
- ✓ Too much potassium can also cause electrolyte imbalances, irregular heartbeats and kidney problems.[22]

In summary, coconut water is a great choice for athletes after strenuous workouts and those who are unwell and experiencing nutrient deficiencies. Both these groups may have an electrolyte shortfall, which can be mitigated by drinking coconut water.

For the average person, though, moderation is key, and coconut water consumption should be limited to a glass a day due to the generally high sodium content in modern diets.

HEALTH BENEFITS

Coconut offers numerous benefits for brain, skin, hair and oral health. It may also contribute to weight loss, possess antimicrobial and antifungal properties and enhance exercise endurance.

Brain-Protective Benefits

Alzheimer's disease, Parkinson's disease, epilepsy and some other neurodegenerative conditions are linked to impaired glucose utilization by brain cells.[23]

When blood glucose is scarce or not usable, the body muscles, heart and liver can utilize fats (free fatty acids) in the blood to generate energy. However, free fatty acids cannot easily cross the blood-brain barrier (BBB) to reach the brain cells. Starved for nutrition, the brain nerve cells malfunction and eventually die.

Coconut oil, when consumed, is converted by the liver into a different type of fuel – ketones. They can pass through the BBB and provide energy to brain cells that cannot process glucose.[24] Coconut oil is believed to protect against many brain disorders by providing an alternate energy source for starving brain cells.

- ✓ Coconut oil may help protect against Alzheimer's disease.[25]
- ✓ It may aid in reducing the frequency of epileptic seizures.[26]

Weight-Loss Benefits

The efficacy of coconut oil for weight loss remains contentious.
- ✓ As a fatty substance, coconut oil is very high in calories. Fats do not typically help in weight loss.
- ✓ The ketones produced from coconut oil may suppress appetite.[27]
- ✓ Some argue that the medium-chain fatty acids in coconut oil could be beneficial for weight loss,[28] but there is no direct evidence to support this claim.

- ✓ When combined with a low-fat diet, coconut oil may enhance fat burning and reduce appetite.[29]

Nevertheless, it is advisable to await more research-based evidence before endorsing coconut oil as a weight-loss aid.

Exercise-Related Benefits

The ability of coconut oil to provide quick energy and boost calorie burn enhances exercise performance, especially among athletes.[30]

We have so far focused on the benefits of ingesting food items, not their topical use. Coconut and its products have a long history of application for skin, hair and oral health, which we'll delve into next.

Skin Health Benefits

- ✓ Coconut oil has antioxidant and anti-inflammatory properties, making it effective for soothing burnt, irritated, infected or inflamed skin.[31]
- ✓ Applying coconut oil to the skin can prevent moisture loss and dryness.[32]
- ✓ Damaged skin loses its protective barrier function, but coconut oil aids in repairing and restoring this function.[33]
- ✓ It can improve wound healing when applied topically.[34]

Note: Coconut oil can block skin pores, so it should not be applied to oily and acne-prone skin.

Hair Health Benefits

Coconut oil has been a trusted hair care remedy for centuries.
- ✓ It penetrates the hair better than most oils,[35] reducing water absorption and preventing cycles of hair swelling and drying, which can lead to breakage.[36]
- ✓ Coconut oil prevents protein loss from hair during washing.[37]
- ✓ The oil can also help control dandruff due to its antifungal (restricting the fungus growth) and anti-inflammatory (soothing scalp irritation) properties.[38]

Antimicrobial Benefits

Coconut oil, powered by lauric acid, offers various antimicrobial benefits:
- ✓ When applied to the skin, it can combat yeast infections like ringworm.[39]
- ✓ For vaginal fungal infections, a tampon coated with coconut oil can be inserted to apply to the infected area.[40] Candida, a common fungus, often causes such infections, leading to inflammation, intense itchiness and white discharge from the vagina. Because of the area's hard-to-reach nature, regular applicators might not be effective, necessitating the tampon method.
- ✓ In cases of oral fungal infection, you can try 'oil pulling', a process that involves swishing about 1 tbsp (15 ml) of coconut oil in the mouth for 15 minutes before spitting it out.[41] Use a teaspoon (5 ml) for children over five. Oil

pulling with coconut oil can improve oral health,[42] and can also be as effective as a conventional mouthwash.[43]

While coconut oil has antibacterial properties, it is not an antibiotic. It cannot replace prescribed medications for killing pathogens. Always follow your doctor's advice for treatment.

HOW TO CONSUME

Here are various ways to consume coconuts:
- ✓ **Whole coconuts**: Easily found in markets, these provide a fresh and nutritious option.
- ✓ **Virgin coconut oil**: This unrefined oil offers a distinct aroma and flavour. It's suitable for low-temperature cooking, with a smoking point of 175°C (350°F).
- ✓ **Refined coconut oil**: Ideal for high-temperature cooking, with a smoking point of up to 200°C (400°F).
- ✓ **Coconut milk**: Widely available in markets, it's commonly used in cooking.
- ✓ **Coconut water**: Often sold by street vendors in many countries. During summer, coconuts tend to have less water and thicker flesh. Opt for unsweetened varieties when purchasing commercially available coconut water.
- ✓ **Coconut flour**: Available in select markets and online, this flour offers a gluten-free alternative for baking.
- ✓ **Copra**: The dried meat of coconut, typically used in tropical cuisines, either in small pieces or shredded.

HOW TO SELECT

✓ Brown and green coconuts are available in the market in their unhusked form. Brown coconuts are fully mature with less water, and green coconuts are younger, with less flesh but more water, typically harvested for their water content.
✓ Avoid husked coconuts with cracked shells, as they may be spoilt.
✓ Select coconuts that feel heavy for their size, indicating a good amount of flesh inside.

HOW TO STORE

✓ Fully de-husked coconuts can be stored at room temperature for about two to three weeks.
✓ Coconuts with an intact husk can be stored for four months at room temperature.[44]
✓ To increase the shelf life of de-husked coconuts:
  1. Leave some husk over the three coconut eyes since that area is prone to decay.[45]
  2. Store de-husked coconut in the fridge, which will extend its life to two months.
✓ Fresh coconut flesh can be kept in the refrigerator for up to a week and frozen for up to three months.
✓ Follow the same storage guidelines as coconut flesh for shredded fresh coconut.
✓ Shredded dried coconut can be kept in an airtight container at room temperature for up to five months.

- ✓ Coconut milk should be refrigerated and consumed within three days.
- ✓ Coconut oil turns into a semi-solid below 25°C (76°F) and liquid above this temperature. So, keep it in a cupboard instead of in a refrigerator.
- ✓ Store coconut flour in an airtight container placed in a cool and dark area.

HOW MUCH TO CONSUME

- ✓ Given the debate surrounding the consumption of saturated fats from coconut, here are two options:
  1. If you follow a modern, highly processed diet or are watching your cholesterol intake and blood levels, have up to **30 g** of fresh coconut flesh meat or **1 tbsp** (**15 ml**) of coconut oil daily, through food or otherwise. Most readers of this book will fall into this category.
  2. If you live in a traditional culture, with a diet full of vegetables, fruits and other unprocessed food, you may have up to **100 g** of fresh coconut meat or **3 tbsp** (**45 ml**) of coconut oil a day.
- ✓ **One** glass (**250 ml**) of coconut water a day. You can exceed this if you are unwell or have engaged in an exhausting physical activity.

HOW MUCH IS TOO MUCH

- ✓ Do not exceed **100 g** of fresh coconut flesh or **3 tbsp** (**45 ml**) of coconut oil a day.
- ✓ Do not exceed **two** glasses (**500 ml**) of coconut water a day except when advised by a doctor.

WHO SHOULD AVOID

- ✓ People who have high cholesterol should consult their doctor before increasing their coconut flesh consumption.
- ✓ People allergic to coconut palm pollen or coconut oil should avoid it.
- ✓ Anyone who feels nauseated on consuming coconut oil.

SUMMARY

Systems and Benefits	Major	Minor
Anti-inflammatory		
Antioxidant		
Bones		
Brain	■	
Cancer		
Diabetes		
Digestive		
Eyes		
Heart		
Immunity		■
Joints		
Liver		
Mental Health		
Pregnancy & Lactation		
Reproductive		
Respiratory		
Skin & Hair	■	

Consumption: **30 g** of fresh coconut meat or **1 tbsp (15 ml)** of coconut oil daily. Additionally, **one** glass **(250 ml)** of coconut water a day.

Excess: Stay under **100 g** of fresh coconut meat or **3 tbsp (45 ml)** of coconut oil daily. Don't exceed **two** glasses **(500 ml)** of coconut water a day.

15

JAMUN
(JAVA PLUM)
Diabetes Defender

Avvaiyar was a celebrated Tamizh poetess and saint in the Sangam period 2,000 years ago.[1] As an ascetic, she spent her life writing devotional poems. Her sayings continue to resonate in Tamizh culture today.

The story goes that Avvaiyar, during one of her journeys from one village to another on foot, found herself tired and hungry. Seeking rest, she saw a young shepherd perched on a jamun tree nearby and requested some fruits from him. He asked her, 'Do you want the fruits hot or cold?' Thinking it was a silly question from an uneducated child, Avvaiyar requested cold fruits. Smiling, the boy shook a few tree branches, causing sweet jamun fruits to fall to the ground. Avvaiyar picked some up and blew air at them to get rid of the dirt. With a twinkle in his eyes, the boy enquired, 'Why are you blowing air at the fruits? Are they hot?'

Avvaiyar realized that the boy had tricked her with his words. Before this encounter, she had believed her knowledge of Tamizh to be second to none, but this boy had humbly reminded her that no matter one's mastery, there is always more to learn.

As she looked up, she saw Lord Murugan – the guardian deity of the Tamizh language and literature – standing in place of the boy. This divine revelation unfolded into a dialogue, with Lord Murugan posing to Avvaiyar deep questions about life and she responding to them. The exchange has come to us as a masterpiece of Tamizh literature, celebrating the power of language and the wisdom of the ages. And somehow, jamuns have played an important role in it.[2]

Jamun (scientific name *Syzygium cumini*) is a prominent tree native to the Indian subcontinent. Every year in the month of May, it yields large oblong berries, whose colour changes from green to crimson to deep purple as they ripen. These berries are characterized by their sweet, sour and astringent flavour.

NUTRIENTS

Jamun Fruit

The jamun fruit has 83 per cent water, 16 per cent carbohydrates, 0.7 per cent proteins and 0.2 per cent fats.[3]

Nutrition in Suggested Daily Amount of Jamun		Eat **100** grams
		Has **60** calories
Source	*Nutrient*	*Daily Need (%)*
Good	*Vitamin C*	17.9
	Magnesium	5.0
Poor	*Dietary Fibres*	4.3
	Phosphorous, vitamin B_6 (pyridoxine), calcium, potassium, vitamin B_3 (niacin), sodium, vitamin B_2 (riboflavin), iron, vitamin B_1 (Thiamine), vitamin A equivalent, vitamin B_5 (pantothenic acid), vitamin B_9 (folate), vitamin E, vitamin K, copper, manganese, selenium and zinc	Less than 3

Aside from vitamin C and magnesium, jamun contains very few other vitamins and minerals, contrary to claims on several popular websites. However, the jamun fruit is rich in many protective plant compounds:[4]

- ✓ **Anthocyanins:** Contain antioxidant, anti-cancer, anti-diabetes and anti-microbial properties, protecting the heart, brain and vision.[5] They are responsible for the purple colour of the fruits.
- ✓ **Ellagic acid:** Antioxidant, anti-inflammatory, anti-cancer and anti-diabetic properties. It also protects the brain, heart, skin and immune system.[6]
- ✓ **Myrecetin:** Antioxidant, anti-cancer, antimicrobial, heart-protecting and anti-diabetic properties[7]
- ✓ **Kaempferol:** Antioxidant, anti-inflammatory, anti-cancer and antimicrobial compound that protects the heart, brain, bones, liver, lungs and digestive system[8]

- ✓ **Isoquercetin:** Antioxidant, anti-inflammatory, anti-cancer, anti-diabetes and anti-allergy properties[9]

Jamun Seeds

The jamun fruit has a single large, hard and tasteless seed at its core, which can be ground into powder for consumption. The data regarding its nutritional profile is all over the place, though. According to reports, its moisture content (water percentage) ranges from 9 to 57 per cent, while its fibre content is anywhere between 1 and 6 per cent![10]

Luckily, the recommended daily intake of jamun seed powder is only 3 to 6 g. So, its vitamins, minerals and fibre contents are insignificant. Nonetheless, jamun seeds contain a few beneficial plant compounds:[11]

- ✓ **Jamboline and jambosine:** These prevent the conversion of starch to glucose,[12] making the powdered form of jamun seeds valuable for diabetes management.
- ✓ **Ellagic acid:** (Refer to compounds listed under the jamun fruit.)

HEALTH BENEFITS

Traditional Benefits

According to Ayurveda, while the jamun fruit enhances the vata dosha, it also balances the kapha and pitta doshas. With its water-absorbing properties, it provides relief from diarrhoea and dysentery. Additionally, it may alleviate throat discomfort, asthma and other respiratory challenges. It improves digestion and addresses issues like tiredness, weight loss and emaciation, and is reportedly effective against infections, worm infestations and an overactive bladder.[13]

Modern Benefits

Jamun provides various health benefits, owing to its antioxidant, anti-inflammatory, antimicrobial, anti-allergic, anti-cancer and anti-diabetic properties. It also protects the digestive system, heart, liver and maintains oral health.[14]

Although the bark and flowers of the jamun tree carry health benefits as well, for the purposes of this discussion, we will focus on the benefits of the fruit and seeds, as these are the ones readily available for purchase.

Antioxidant and Anti-Inflammatory Benefits

- ✓ Many of the antioxidant compounds found in jamun help prevent free radical damage and degeneration in the body.[15]
- ✓ Jamun also exhibits anti-inflammatory properties.[16]

Anti-Diabetic Benefits

Jamun is renowned for its anti-diabetic properties.[17] Before the advent of insulin, it was a key component of diabetes treatment, operating through several mechanisms:[18]

- ✓ The seeds contain compounds that slow down starch digestion into glucose.[19] This helps in managing diabetes and obesity.[20]
- ✓ It improves the function of insulin in patients who have high blood glucose levels.[21]
- ✓ It lowers average blood glucose in diabetic patients whose blood glucose remain elevated despite proper diet and medication.[22]
- ✓ Additionally, jamun may also offer protection against common diabetic complications such as heart and liver damage.[23]

- ✓ Some research papers claim that jamun seeds are high in dietary fibre, which, in theory, can slow down the absorption of blood glucose in the intestines.[24] But that cannot hold true since the suggested dose of jamun seed powder is too little to contain much fibre.

Digestive Benefits

- ✓ The antioxidants present in jamun may prevent oxidative stress and free radical damage in the intestines. This may prevent digestive disorders such as ulcerative colitis and gastritis.
- ✓ Jamun stimulates bile production, which helps us digest fats.
- ✓ Consuming jamun powder may reduce the risk of developing gastric ulcers and aid in their healing process. The seeds contain compounds that help reduce stomach acid and boost the protective mucus lining of the stomach.[25]
- ✓ Its astringent properties may alleviate chronic diarrhoea.[26]
- ✓ Jamun's carminative properties can provide relief from issues related to gas.
- ✓ Contrary to common belief, jamun fruit contains too little dietary fibre to address constipation.

Heart-Protective Benefits

- ✓ Jamun seeds may improve the blood cholesterol profile.[27]
- ✓ They may also increase antioxidant enzymes in heart muscles.[28]
- ✓ Jamun seed powder is found to lower blood pressure by up to 35 per cent.[29] This benefit is likely due to its ellagic acid content.

- ✓ Consuming the flesh of the jamun fruit may prevent rise in blood pressure in chronically stressed individuals.[30]

Respiratory Benefits

- ✓ Jamun seed compounds have antiviral properties. They can protect the body from respiratory infections.[31]
- ✓ The vitamin C in jamun fruit can improve lung function by reducing inflammation in the airways.

Anti-Cancer Benefits

Many compounds in jamun have anti-cancer properties:[32]

- ✓ Antioxidants in jamun, such as anthocyanins, ellagic acid, myrecetin, kaempferol and vitamin C, protect the body from oxidative damage that can lead to the formation of cancer cells.
- ✓ Jamun may help stop the spread of cancer as anthocyanins are recognized for preventing cancer cell growth or killing them.

The research on jamun's anti-cancer properties is still in its early stages. The prudent approach would be to enjoy jamun for its potential benefits but never to solely depend on it for cancer treatment.

Antimicrobial Benefits

- ✓ Jamun possesses antibacterial and antifungal properties.[33]
- ✓ It can eliminate harmful bacteria in the intestines while preserving the beneficial ones.[34] This is significant because antibiotics are known to indiscriminately kill gut bacteria, including the helpful ones.[35]

But this should not discourage you from your prescribed

antibiotic treatment. Instead, consider consuming jamun fruit or its seed powder to boost your body's immunity.

Anti-Anaemic Benefits

Several websites and research papers claim that jamun has high iron content, thereby improving blood iron and haemoglobin levels.[36]

However, note that 100 g of jamun, the typical daily portion, just contains 0.19 mg of iron, whereas young women are advised to intake 29 mg of iron per day. So, it can only provide 0.7 per cent of the daily requirement, making it a poor source of iron.

A potential counterargument could be that jamun is high in vitamin C, which helps improve iron absorption. But given the little iron in jamun to start with, how much can you additionally absorb? There are no research trials addressing this. As the saying goes, 'when in doubt, stay out'.

HOW TO CONSUME

- ✓ Jamun can be enjoyed raw. But it can leave stains on your lips, tongue and clothing if you're not careful.
- ✓ These fruits have a sour, tangy and slightly sweet taste. A pinch of salt can enhance their flavour.
- ✓ You can incorporate the jamun flesh into smoothies, fruit bowls and sorbets.
- ✓ It can be juiced into punches, mocktails and cocktails.
- ✓ Consider making jamun jams, jellies, syrups and desserts such as cakes, puddings, mousse, fruit yoghurts and ice creams.
- ✓ It also pairs well with various foods and flavours, including mangoes, grapes, strawberries, cucumber, ginger, mint,

cinnamon, honey, yoghurt, coconut milk and honey.[37]

HOW TO SELECT

- ✓ Jamun fruits are picked when they are ripe and dark purple. They are never artificially ripened.
- ✓ Try to avoid green, unripe fruits.
- ✓ Freshly picked jamun fruits will usually have their stems attached.
- ✓ Select fruits with intact skin, free of bruises or soft spots. A juicy jamun should feel relatively heavy for its size, with a sweet aroma.
- ✓ A light, dried fruit with shrivelled skin is likely past its prime.
- ✓ If jamun is mushy with a sour scent, it may be overripe and depleted of nutrients.
- ✓ As a seasonal fruit, jamun is best eaten as a fresh fruit, but its pulp, juice, dried powder or tablets can be consumed during the rest of the year.
- ✓ Various products extracted from its fruit, seed, bark and flower are available for medicinal use.

HOW TO STORE

- ✓ For optimal taste, consume ripe jamuns the same day after harvesting.
- ✓ Ripe fruits can last in the fridge for up to two weeks if stored in paper or plastic wrap, although this may result in an inferior flavour.
- ✓ Avoid storing jamun with apples or bananas, as the latter emit ethylene gas that can overripen jamun fruits, spoiling them.

HOW MUCH TO CONSUME

- ✓ A typical jamun fruit weighs 10 to 20 g.[38] The seed is usually around 2 g.
- ✓ Eat around **100 g** of fresh jamun fruits a day to enjoy its health benefits. Given their seasonal availability, however, one should consider other forms for regular use.
- ✓ Do not consume jamun fruit on an empty stomach, as it is highly acidic. Eat it with other food.
- ✓ Avoid jamun fruit one hour before or after drinking milk or milk-based beverages.
- ✓ Do not consume unripe jamun fruit, as it contains high levels of toxins that can lead to a stomach upset and diarrhoea.
- ✓ Alternatively, you can drink **4 tsp** (**20 ml**) of jamun juice alongside your breakfast.
- ✓ For managing blood glucose, consume **1 tsp** (**6 g**) of jamun seed powder per day instead of fresh fruits or juice. It is best to divide this amount into two equal doses of 3 g each to be taken with lunch and dinner. Should you divide it into three doses of 2 g each if you have three meals daily? Logically, yes!

HOW MUCH IS TOO MUCH

- ✓ No toxic levels have been established for jamun consumption.
- ✓ Excessive intake may lead to constipation, acne breakouts and vomiting.

- ✓ It is recommended to limit intake to no more than **100 g** of fresh jamun fruits, **4 tsp** of jamun juice or **6 g** of jamun seed powder.

WHO SHOULD AVOID

- ✓ Jamun lowers blood glucose levels, so diabetics taking blood glucose-lowering medicines should be careful of hypoglycaemia if they take both together.
- ✓ Pregnant and lactating women should avoid excessive consumption of jamun, as its effects on a foetus or a newborn through breast milk have not been studied.
- ✓ According to Ayurveda, jamun increases the vata dosha in the body. Thus, people with symptoms of increased vata, such as dry, rough skin or lips, bloating, constipation, weight loss, dehydration, dizziness, muscle twitching, anxiety, agitation, restlessness, palpitations or inability to get proper sleep, should steer clear of it.[39]

SUMMARY

Systems and Benefits	Major	Minor
Anti-inflammatory		■
Antioxidant	■	
Bones		
Brain		
Cancer		■
Diabetes	■	
Digestive	■	
Eyes		
Heart	■	
Immunity		■
Joints		
Liver		
Mental Health		
Pregnancy & Lactation		
Reproductive		
Respiratory		■
Skin & Hair		

Consumption: Either **100 g** of fresh fruits, **4 tsp (20 ml)** of juice or **1 tsp (6 g)** of seed powder.

Excess: Avoid exceeding these quantities.

16

CAPSICUM
(BELL PEPPERS)
Heart Protector

Christopher Columbus returned to Europe from Central America in 1493, bringing along a variety of peppers. Some of them were spicy, while others – characterized by their red, yellow and green colours – were milder and sweeter. Oddly enough, these gentler peppers remained relatively unknown in Europe for the next four centuries for an interesting reason.

The sweet peppers were hollow with thin, hard walls. Within each pepper was a long stick-like structure – the remnant of the flower's stigma, the outermost part that produces a sweet scent to attract pollinating insects. As these peppers swayed in the wind, this piece would knock against the wall, generating a chime-like sound that earned them their 'bell' pepper moniker. The sound frightened off grazing livestock and disrupted the villagers' sleep at night, making it a challenging crop to cultivate.

Luckily, Gregor Carillon, a plant breeder in Szeged, Hungary, decided to develop a silent bell pepper. On 1 April 1908, he unveiled the world's first 'quiet' bell pepper, which gained rapid popularity.[1] Despite its silence, the 'bell pepper' label has stuck, with many justifying it by pointing to the pepper's bell-like appearance.

Capsicums are fruits belonging to the nightshade family, like eggplants and tomatoes. Bell peppers (scientific name *Capsicum annuum*) are a type of capsicum, a genus that includes chilli peppers, their hotter and spicier cousins. Sweeter in taste, bell peppers are also called sweet peppers. While chilli peppers are native to Central America, bell peppers are grown all over the world because of their ability to thrive in warm weather and moist soil.

The term 'bell peppers' is common in the US, Canada and the Philippines, while in the UK and South Africa, they are just called 'peppers' or 'sweet peppers'. In India, Pakistan, Bangladesh, Sri Lanka, Malaysia, Australia and New Zealand, they are known as 'capsicum'.

The word capsicum derives from the Latin *capsa*, meaning a box, due to the fruit's distinctive square shape. This chapter focuses on bell peppers, which we will refer to as capsicums – their Indian name.

These fruits come in a variety of colours based on individual plant pigments. Common colours include green, yellow, orange and red, but they also appear in shades of brown, white and purple.[2] Typically, these strains are named according to their colours, i.e., red peppers or yellow capsicums.

All varieties share a characteristic tangy taste paired with a crunchy texture. The green and purple peppers are slightly bitter, while the ones in red, yellow and orange are known for their sweetness.

NUTRIENTS

Red capsicums contain 92 per cent water, 6.7 per cent carbohydrates, 0.9 per cent proteins and 0.1 per cent fats.[3]

Nutrition in Suggested Daily Amount of **Capsicum**		Eat **150 grams**
		Has **41 calories**
Source	*Nutrient*	*Daily Need (%)*
Great	*Vitamin C*	266.3
	Vitamin B_9 (Folate)	35.3
	Vitamin E	23.7
	Vitamin A equivalent	23.6
	Vitamin B_6 (pyridoxine)	22.5
	Vitamin K	20.2
Good	*Vitamin B_2 (riboflavin)*	13.3
	Vitamin B_5 (pantothenic acid)	9.5
	Selenium	9.4
	Manganese	9.2
	Vitamin B_3 (niacin)	8.3
	Dietary Fibres	6.8
	Potassium	6.8
	Phosphorous	6.8
	Vitamin B_1 (thiamine)	5.9
	Magnesium	5.5
Poor	*Copper, iron, zinc, calcium and sodium*	Less than 3

✓ Capsicums offer a wide range of vitamins and minerals, unlike other superfoods that are predominantly rich only in a few nutrients.

- ✓ Different capsicums boast varying nutrient profiles. For example, compared to their green counterparts, red capsicums provide twice the amount of vitamin C and eight times the vitamin A.[4]

These peppers also contain beneficial plant compounds:[5]
- ✓ **Quercetin:**[6] Exhibits antioxidant,[7] anti-inflammatory,[8] anti-allergic,[9] anti-cancer,[10] brain-protective[11] and heart-protective properties[12]
- ✓ **Lutein and Zeaxanthin:** Found in green capsicums. They have antioxidant, anti-inflammatory and anti-cancer properties, and protect the eyes, heart and brain.[13]
- ✓ **Lycopene:** Antioxidant, anti-inflammatory, anti-cancer and anti-diabetes properties. It also protects the heart, brain, bones, eyes and skin.[14] Though some experts claim that red capsicums do not contain lycopene,[15] evidence shows they do.[16] In fact, 150 g of cooked red peppers will offer 700 μg of lycopene, amounting to around 7 per cent of the daily recommended amount.
- ✓ **Luteolin:** Antioxidant, anti-inflammatory, anti-allergic, anti-cancer and heart-protective properties.[17]
- ✓ **Capsiate:** Contributes to the management of heart disease, cancers, digestive disorders, metabolic disorders and obesity.[18]

Caution: The Internet is filled with websites (and even research papers!) attributing the numerous benefits of bell peppers to a 'miracle' ingredient – capsaicin. However, bell peppers contain capsiate, not capsaicin. Chilli peppers are famous for their capsaicin, a compound that causes burning sensation in the mouth.

HEALTH BENEFITS

Capsicums may help prevent and manage diabetes, heart disease and cancers, while also boosting immunity, protecting vision and promoting wound healing.[19]

Heart-Protective Benefits

- ✓ Being rich in vitamins B_6 and B_9, capsicums help reduce blood levels of a protein called homocysteine, which, at elevated levels, can damage the inner lining of blood vessels and increase the risk of blood clot formation.[20]
- ✓ The dietary fibres in capsicums can minimize cholesterol absorption in the intestines.
- ✓ Capsicums contain compounds that inhibit fat digestion.[21] An enzyme in the intestines breaks down dietary fats into fatty acids, which are then absorbed into the blood. However, capsicums block this action, thereby decreasing the amount of absorbable fatty acids in the intestines. Yellow and red peppers are particularly effective for this, followed by green ones.
- ✓ Red peppers are beneficial for heart health due to their lycopene content, a potent antioxidant.[22]
- ✓ Capsicums are also rich in the antioxidant vitamins A, C and E, all of which contribute to protecting the heart.

Anti-Diabetes Benefits

- ✓ Predominantly composed of water, capsicums present a healthy, low-calorie option for diabetic diets.
- ✓ Being an excellent source of dietary fibre, capsicums

slow down glucose absorption in the intestines. They help prevent large blood glucose spikes after meals. This fibre also maintains satiety for extended periods, curbing hunger pangs between meals.
- ✓ Compounds in capsicums can reduce carbohydrate digestion.[23] An enzyme in the intestines breaks down dietary carbohydrates into glucose, which is then absorbed into the bloodstream. Capsicums block this enzymatic action, resulting in less glucose being available for absorption. Yellow peppers are particularly efficient in this regard, followed by red and green peppers.
- ✓ Antioxidants in capsicums may protect against type 2 diabetes and its harmful long-term complications, such as heart disease and retinal damage.[24]

Anti-Cancer Benefits

The antioxidant and anti-inflammatory compounds in capsicum offer protection against cancer[25] by combatting chronic oxidative stress and excessive inflammation – two factors that can increase the risk of cancers.
- ✓ Capsicums are rich in carotenoids that have many cancer-related benefits.[26]
- ✓ Certain sulphur-containing compounds in capsicums also protect against cancer.[27]
- ✓ Capsicums contain dietary fibres that reduce the risk of certain cancers.[28]
- ✓ The lycopene in red capsicum is known to protect against cancers of the cervix, bladder, prostate and pancreas through various mechanisms.[29]

- ✓ The capsiate in capsicums plays many preventive roles in the development of cancer.[30]

Eye-Protective Benefits

- ✓ Capsicums are abundant in antioxidants, lutein and zeaxanthin, which protect the eyes from the risk of developing age-related cataracts and macular degeneration.[31]
- ✓ They serve as excellent sources of antioxidant vitamins A, C and E, protecting against the same eye conditions.[32]

HOW TO CONSUME

- ✓ Capsicums can be enjoyed raw, grilled, roasted, stir-fried, sautéed, baked or pickled. They can also form tasty additions to salads, stews and soups.
- ✓ They pair well with foods such as rice, tomatoes, corn, chickpeas, black beans, fish and poultry.
- ✓ They also complement basil, coriander, parsley, garlic, onions, vinegar, olive oil and various cheeses.[33]
- ✓ Lightly cooking capsicums helps release healthy compounds from their fibrous content, making them easier to absorb. Stir-frying is an ideal cooking method.
- ✓ Deep frying or high-temperature cooking can result in the loss of some vitamin C and delicate antioxidants.

HOW TO SELECT

- ✓ Look for capsicums with a shiny, firm skin and deep colour. Avoid ones with wrinkled skin, soft, watery spots, sunken areas, cuts or brown spots.

- ✓ The stem of capsicum should be fresh and green. Capsicums with dried stems may have sat on the shelf for a while, potentially losing their nutrients.
- ✓ A good-quality capsicum will feel heavy for its size.
- ✓ Capsicums are available all year around.
- ✓ Green capsicums are usually the cheapest option.

HOW TO STORE

- ✓ If you want to store capsicums for later use, do not wash them. Instead, put them in a plastic bag in the refrigerator, where they will stay fresh for a week.
- ✓ For leftover uncooked capsicum pieces, keep them in a plastic bag and refrigerate. They will last for two to three days.
- ✓ Yellow and red capsicums are more delicate and spoil faster than green ones.

HOW MUCH TO CONSUME

While there is no universally recommended amount for capsicum consumption, moderation is always advisable. Experts suggest incorporating **one** medium (**150 g**) capsicum into your daily diet.

HOW MUCH IS TOO MUCH

There are no established guidelines for excess capsicum consumption; nonetheless, overeating capsicum may lead to an unbalanced intake of other healthy vegetables. So, limit your consumption to under **three** medium to large capsicums (**500 g**) daily.

WHO SHOULD AVOID

- ✓ Capsicums are very well tolerated in the amounts typically consumed as food.
- ✓ Those with a pollen allergy may need to be exercise caution while consuming capsicum.[34]
- ✓ When researching online about capsicums, be diligent in verifying the recommended intake, excess doses, side effects and those who should avoid them. As mentioned, many Western sources refer to capsicums as chilli peppers, which require different precautionary measures due to their capsaicin content.[35] In contrast, bell peppers contain capsiate, a different and less pungent substance.

SUMMARY

Systems and Benefits	Major	Minor
Anti-inflammatory		■
Antioxidant	■	
Bones		
Brain		
Cancer	■	
Diabetes	■	
Digestive		
Eyes	■	
Heart	■	
Immunity		
Joints		
Liver		
Mental Health		
Pregnancy & Lactation		
Reproductive		
Respiratory		
Skin & Hair		

Consumption: One medium capsicum (**150 g**) a day.

Excess: Don't consume more than **three** medium to large capsicums (**500 g**) per day.

17

ASAFOETIDA
(HING)
Digestive Powerhouse

In 631 BCE, a group of European settlers relocated to Cyrene, an oasis in present-day Libya.[1] Unique to this region was a hitherto unknown shrub that would make Cyrene the wealthiest city in Africa – silphium.

The delicious, fragrant sap of silphium was laden with medicinal and culinary properties. The Greeks used it to treat cough, sore throat, fever, indigestion, warts, aches and pains. Esteemed culinary experts of the land seasoned their dishes with its grated dry sap and its flowers yielded a delicate perfume. The juice of the silphium plant was known for its aphrodisiac properties.

With the silphium trade, the Cyrenian economy boomed.[2] The Greeks wrote poems about the plant and the Romans composed songs in its praise.[3]

Except for one issue: The plant could only grow in a narrow strip surrounding Cyrene. Soon, human greed took over. People began overharvesting silphium and its price skyrocketed, prompting theft. Counterfeiters duplicated silphium after discovering an herb in Parthia, in modern-day Iran, with similar health and culinary benefits, but also an offensive odour. The crooks started adulterating the resin of silphium with a stinky goo from this variety.

By 96 BCE, silphium stocks had become scarce. Finally, in 60 CE, the last known silphium plant was plucked and presented to Emperor Nero of Rome. With that, one of the most important culinary and medicinal plants went extinct.[4] Without silphium trade, Cyrene faded into obscurity, first as a deserted city and eventually falling into ruin.[5] In time, the world forgot about silphium.

But fake silphium continued to be traded in Parthia. While the original herb had captured European fascination, Persian and Afghan traders were selling the cheaper variety to Indians. Slowly, the foul-smelling resin permeated Indian cuisine and found its way into Ayurvedic medicine. It even ascended to the highest levels of Indian society, where it became a part of religious rituals.[6]

Thus, from Cyrene, Parthia and then to India, the legend of silphium lives on in every Indian kitchen through its ersatz version: asafoetida.

Asafoetida is a dried gum resin extracted from an herb known as *Ferula asafoetida*. These plants are native to Iran, Afghanistan and Central Asia. They typically thrive in arid regions at higher altitudes. Various species of this herb have specific climate preferences, making them difficult to cultivate elsewhere.

NUTRIENTS

Asafoetida contains 16 per cent water, 72 per cent carbohydrates, 4 per cent protein, 1 per cent fats and 7 per cent minerals.[7]

Nutrition in Suggested Daily Amount of **Asafoetida**	Eat **0.5 grams**
	Has **1** calorie
Source *Nutrient*	*Daily Need (%)*
Poor *All vitamins, minerals and dietary fibres*	Less than 3

Asafoetida has plant compounds that offer health benefits even when present in small amounts:[8]

- ✓ **Sulphur compounds:** These have antioxidant, anti-inflammatory, anti-cancer and antimicrobial properties.[9] They are also responsible for the distinctive 'bacterial decomposition' odour of asafoetida.
- ✓ **Phenolic compounds:** These possess antioxidant, anti-inflammatory, anti-cancer and anti-ageing benefits.[10]

HEALTH BENEFITS

Asafoetida is known for its medicinal properties in many cultures and countries around the world.

Traditional Medicinal Uses

It has been used to treat flatulence, stomach ache, poor digestion, digestive system parasites and respiratory conditions such as asthma, bronchitis and whooping cough.[11]

In Ayurveda, asafoetida is known for its carminative (relieving flatulence), digestive and anti-bloating properties. It serves as a cardiac tonic, improves vision and alleviates abdominal colic pain, worm infestation, constipation, abdominal tumours and ascites.[12]

Modern Medicinal Uses

Over the last fifty years, extensive research has been carried out to study the medicinal uses of asafoetida. It contains many beneficial compounds which have antioxidant, antimicrobial, digestive, anti-cancer, anti-diabetes, neuroprotective and heart-protective properties.[13]

Digestive Benefits

Asafoetida frequently features in commercially available digestive powders.
- ✓ It promotes movement of food through the digestive system, alleviating flatulence, which is asafoetida's main claim to fame. Some stardom!
- ✓ Asafoetida is known to boost the secretion of saliva for better digestion of carbohydrates.
- ✓ It stimulates enzymes that help in protein digestion.[14]
- ✓ It enhances bile production in the liver, aiding fat digestion.
- ✓ Asafoetida amplifies activities of digestive enzymes in the pancreas and small intestine.[15]
- ✓ It can offer relief from stomach cramps and abdominal pain. Some of its compounds help relax the digestive tract muscles, reducing stomach spasms.
- ✓ It can mitigate digestive problems such as bloating, post-meal fullness and motion sickness.[16]

- ✓ Asafoetida may also help alleviate symptoms of irritable bowel syndrome, which causes stomach pain, bloating and flatulence.[17]

Heart-Protective Benefits

- ✓ Asafoetida potentially helps in lowering blood pressure[18] by relaxing the muscles that line your blood arteries and allowing them to expand if the blood pressure tries to rise, thereby easing off the increase.
- ✓ It acts as a blood thinner and slows down blood clotting.[19]

Women's Health Benefits

If you experience menstrual pain, heavy flow or irregular periods, consider incorporating asafoetida into your diet. The female hormone progesterone plays an important role in the menstrual cycle. Ovulation occurs on day fourteen, and an egg is released from the ovary. This also causes the release of progesterone, which prepares the body for pregnancy by building the inner lining of the womb. If the egg fails to fertilize, the production of progesterone drops, causing the womb lining to break down and triggering menstrual bleeding.

If progesterone levels are too low, it can lead to long, heavy periods or irregular bleeding.[20] Asafoetida stimulates progesterone production, helping control menstrual irregularities.

Brain-Protective Benefits

- ✓ It improves learning and memory,[21] benefits attributed to its antioxidant properties.
- ✓ With its sulphur-containing compounds, it aids in preventing memory loss.[22]

- ✓ Asafoetida might also help reduce the occurrence of epileptic seizures, an effect potentially resulting from its ability to lower oxidative stress. A key player in the development of epilepsy is oxidative damage, which can degrade brain nerve cells, rewire brain circuits, increase excitability and induce seizures even in response to minor triggers.[23]

Nerve-Protective Benefits

- ✓ Renowned as a nerve stimulant, asafoetida is useful in therapies for various neurological disorders.[24]
- ✓ The herb helps heal damaged peripheral nerves – those outside the brain and spinal cord.[25] If injured, they can cause peripheral neuropathy, a condition manifesting as numbness, pain and weakness, usually in the hands and feet. But it can also affect digestion and urination.

  Can asafoetida help patients suffering from peripheral neuropathy caused by long-term diabetes? Unfortunately, no studies have directly explored this benefit, but it is logically possible. There is no harm in considering asafoetida consumption for this purpose: heads, you win; tails, you don't lose.

Mental Health Benefits

Asafoetida has shown anxiolytic (anxiety-reducing), analgesic and sedative properties, depending on the dose:[26]

- ✓ In low doses, asafoetida can replace anxiolytic medicines that are used for mild anxiety.
- ✓ In high doses, asafoetida may be a better alternative to current medications such as diazepam for severe anxiety disorders.

It does not have the side effects of many anti-anxiety medicines. But please do not suspend your treatment because there are serious consequences to discontinuing your anxiety medicines abruptly. Add asafoetida to your diet and see if it bolsters your current treatment.

Anti-Cancer Benefits

- ✓ It has anti-cancer and tumour-reducing properties.[27]
- ✓ Asafoetida may also help against the cancers of the ovaries,[28] breast[29] and liver[30].

However, you must follow your doctor's treatment. Asafoetida can be added to your diet to strengthen your battle against cancer.

Liver-Protective Benefits

In a damaged liver, the blood levels of various enzymes become erratic. Asafoetida can significantly reduce the elevated levels of liver enzymes.[31]

Anti-Microbial Benefits

Asafoetida exhibits many antiviral,[32] antibacterial[33] and antifungal[34] properties.

Diabetes-Protective Benefits

It can lower blood glucose levels because of its phenolic acid and tannin compounds.[35]

Fertility Benefits

Asafoetida may boost sperm count and viability.[36] So it could be beneficial in treating low sperm conditions like oligozoospermia.

Respiratory Benefits

- ✓ Asafoetida may relieve asthma symptoms by relaxing the bronchial muscles that line the lung airways, which become inflamed and constricted, causing breathing difficulties.[37]
- ✓ Even in traditional medicine, asafoetida has been used to treat asthma and bronchitis.

HOW TO CONSUME

Asafoetida is mainly consumed through food, though it is also found in some digestive powders, and, on rare occasions, in dietary supplements.

Resin

The thick carrot-like roots of asafoetida plant are scoured to release a milky sap. This sap solidifies into a gummy mass and turns dark brown when dried, forming lumps of pure asafoetida available in wholesale markets.

Powder

The pure lumps are difficult to grate into powder form, which is essential for better portion control in cooking. Moreover, they have a powerful odour and flavour. So, they are mixed with rice or wheat flour before being ground into a fine powder. This asafoetida powder, available in retail stores, typically contains 40 per cent asafoetida, unlike the pure resin form.

Asafoetida Water or Tea

- ✓ Dissolve a dash of asafoetida in a glass of water and add a pinch of rock salt.
- ✓ You can also infuse warm ginger tea with asafoetida and rock salt as both of them help with digestive health.

Asafoetida is widely used in Indian, Pakistani and Middle Eastern cuisines, but here are some tips for using it correctly:

- ✓ Do not add it to your food like salt.
- ✓ It is recommended to fry it in hot oil, butter or ghee (clarified butter) for a few seconds. This process, known as *tadka* in north Indian cooking, reduces its bitterness, mellows its flavour and boosts aroma when added during cooking.
- ✓ Since pulses and beans are highly fibrous, they can cause flatulence, bloating and stomach discomfort. Adding asafoetida to such dishes can improve digestion.
- ✓ Despite its bitterness, asafoetida in small quantities acts as a flavour enhancer. Its sulphurous compounds add flavour to savoury dishes, subtly mimicking garlic, onions and eggs.

The Fifth Taste

For a long time, food scientists categorized four primary flavours: sweet, salty, sour and bitter. All others were considered a combination of these. Recently, however, a fifth, a taste that cannot be replicated by a mixture of the original four, has been recognized. It is called *umami*, translating to 'essence of deliciousness' in Japanese.

> Umami is closely linked to the taste of ajinomoto or monosodium glutamate (MSG), a salt that imparts a savoury, meaty flavour. Asafoetida is recognized for its ability to contribute an umami taste to food.

HOW TO SELECT

- Asafoetida comes in two main varieties: milky white (*hing kabuli sufaid*) and red (*hing lal*). Their flavours are slightly different, with the former being water-soluble and the latter oil-soluble.[38]
- When asafoetida resin is processed into powder, it is mixed with wheat flour in north India and rice flour in the South.
- If you have a sensitivity to gluten, it's crucial to check the label on the asafoetida container and choose products made from rice flour.
- Check the expiry date before buying, as asafoetida loses its volatile oils and pungency quickly. It's best to avoid buying asafoetida powder that is close to its expiration date.
- You can get asafoetida in bricket, tablet or free-flowing powder forms. The powder form is the easiest for kitchen use.
- It is probably the most adulterated food ingredient in the market, usually mixed with inferior-grade asafoetida or red clay, sand, stones and gypsum.[39] Though it is difficult to detect a lower-grade asafoetida as an adulterant, there are two tests to identify other kinds of potential adulteration:[40]

1. Take a small amount of asafoetida in a spoon and burn it. Pure asafoetida will burn with a flame like camphor, while adulterated resin barely produces a flame.
2. Dissolve a little asafoetida is a glass of lukewarm water. Mix it thoroughly and let it settle. Pure asafoetida will result in a milky white solution with no sediments. In contrast, adulterated asafoetida will leave tiny stones or earthy matter at the bottom.

To avoid the risk of adulteration, opt for a trusted brand.

HOW TO STORE

✓ Place in an airtight container unless you want your neighbours to know about your secret ingredient, as its smell can pervade your home. Even inside your spice cabinet, a loosely closed lid will lend asafoetida's 'aroma' to all other spices.

✓ Once you've used a container for storing asafoetida, do not try to repurpose it for anything else, as the smell will linger long after the powder is finished.

HOW MUCH TO CONSUME

There is no recommended daily dose of asafoetida. However, 200 to 500 mg per day of asafoetida resin in its pure form is the quantity used traditionally for medicinal purposes.[41] The powder you get in the market has only 40 per cent resin. So, aim to consume **500** to **1,250 mg** of asafoetida powder daily for its health benefits.

HOW MUCH IS TOO MUCH

- Up to **500 mg** a day of pure asafoetida or **1,250 mg** of asafoetida powder has been found to cause no harm.[42] Do not exceed these amounts.
- Too much asafoetida can cause swelling in the mouth, flatulence, diarrhoea, anxiety, headaches and bleeding problems.[43]

WHO SHOULD AVOID

- Pregnant women should avoid consuming asafoetida in large amounts,[44] as it can lead to miscarrying.[45] While the amount in food is generally safe, it's advisable to steer clear of asafoetida water.
- Breastfeeding women should especially exercise caution since foetuses possess a different type of haemoglobin than adults in the blood. Given that they get oxygen from their mother's blood – a poor source – and not from the air, the foetal haemoglobin is designed to carry more oxygen.[46] Many compounds in asafoetida strongly oxidize haemoglobin, converting it into a compound called methaemoglobin, which lacks the ability to bind and transport oxygen around the body. While it poses no harm to adults, infants can face life-threatening situations due to their distinct haemoglobin.[47] Since these oxidizing compounds pass through breast milk to the nursing infant, breastfeeding mothers should limit their consumption of asafoetida. Interestingly, within six months of birth, an infant's haemoglobin is gradually replaced by the adult type.[48] So, breastfeeding mothers can safely consume

asafoetida after this period.
- ✓ Since asafoetida lowers blood glucose, it's crucial to monitor your blood glucose levels to prevent hypoglycaemia if you consume diabetes medication.
- ✓ Asafoetida contains toxic compounds called coumarins, which have blood-thinning properties. If you are on blood-thinning medicines, moderate your asafoetida consumption.
- ✓ If you are planning to undergo a surgery, it's wise to halt any overconsumption of asafoetida two weeks before and after the procedure to minimize the chances of excess bleeding.
- ✓ Gluten-sensitive people should avoid asafoetida mixed with wheat flour. Opt for the rice flour-blended version.

SUMMARY

Systems and Benefits	Major	Minor
Anti-inflammatory		■
Antioxidant		■
Bones		
Brain		■
Cancer		■
Diabetes		■
Digestive	■	
Eyes		
Heart		■
Immunity		■
Joints		
Liver		■
Mental Health		■
Pregnancy & Lactation		
Reproductive	■	
Respiratory		■
Skin & Hair		

Consumption: 200 to **500 mg** of pure resin or **500** to **1,250 mg** of powder daily.

Excess: Strictly avoid for infants. Avoid more than **500 mg** of pure resin or **1,250 mg** of powder daily.

18

MORINGA
(DRUMSTICKS)
Antioxidant All-Rounder

In 327 BCE, after conquering the Achaemenid empire of Persia, Alexander the Great set his sights on India.¹ His armies started moving eastwards, sweeping through Kabul and Kunar in Afghanistan, followed by Panjkora, Swat and Aornus in Pakistan. Upon crossing the Jhelum river, they defeated King Porus and the Pauravas.² This encounter also brought them into direct conflict with the Mauryan empire across the Ganga.

The folklore goes that the ancient Mauryan warriors drank an extract of moringa leaves every day, which gave them superhuman strength. As a result, they needed little sleep, rarely got sick and the pain from their battle injuries was easily numbed. Roman historians would describe the Mauryan fighters as 'men of stamina and valour'. Over the next two years, these soldiers pounded Alexander's armies in dozens of skirmishes. Dejected and frustrated, Alexander turned back to his native Macedonia and died soon after in Babylon, in 323 BCE.

What an incredible story praising the virtues of moringa and its leaf juice! Except for a minor detail.

Chandragupta Maurya established his empire five years after Alexander the Great left India. There was no way his fighters could have clashed with Alexander's army. It was the latter's enormous losses in the battle of Hyaspes (Jhelum) against King Porus, not the power of moringa, that had forced forced him to head home.[3]

But why should facts get in the way of a great story?

Moringa (scientific name: *Moringa oleifera*) is a plant native to the Indian subcontinent. It is grown as a vegetable and used as an ingredient in traditional medicines. Most parts of the moringa plant, including its leaves, seeds, bark, roots, sap and flowers, have beneficial properties, earning it the moniker of 'miracle plant'. It is also referred to as the 'drumstick tree' due to the shape of its seed pods.

NUTRIENTS

Moringa Leaves

The most nutritious part of the moringa tree are its leaves. They contain 79 per cent water, 8.3 per cent carbohydrates, 9.4 per cent proteins and 1.4 per cent fats.[4]

Nutrition in Suggested Daily Amount of **Moringa Leaves**		Eat **60 grams**
		Has **36 calories**
Source	*Nutrient*	*Daily Need (%)*
Great	Vitamin C	38.8
	Vitamin B_6 (pyridoxine)	36.0
	Magnesium	29.4
	Vitamin B_2 (riboflavin)	24.8
	Vitamin A equivalent	22.7
Good	Vitamin B_9 (folate)	12.0
	Phosphorous	11.2
	Calcium	11.1
	Manganese	11.1
	Vitamin B_1 (thiamine)	11.0
	Iron	8.3
	Vitamin B_3 (niacin)	7.4
Poor	Potassium	4.3
	Copper	3.2
	Dietary Fibres	3.0
	Zinc, vitamin B_5 (pantothenic acid), selenium, sodium, vitamin E and vitamin K	Less than 3

Some cautionary details are due:

✓ 60 g of moringa leaves contain 5.6 g of plant protein. Unfortunately, this protein is poorly absorbed in the intestines.[5] So, do not count on moringa leaves to augment your protein intake, contrary to what some experts claim.[6]

✓ Moringa leaves contain compounds called tannins and oxalates, which tightly bind to calcium and iron.[7] Once attached to these compounds, the two minerals cannot be absorbed in the intestines and are eliminated through the stools. As a result, while the moringa leaves contain a good amount of calcium and iron, our bodies get very little from eating them. This is why tannins and oxalates are called anti-nutrients.

Moringa Seed Pods (Drumsticks)

The fruits of the moringa tree are its seed pods. They have 88 per cent water, 8.5 per cent carbohydrates, 2.1 per cent proteins and 0.2 per cent fats.[8]

Nutrition in Suggested Daily Amount of **Moringa Seed Pods**		Eat **100** grams
		Has **37** calories
Source	*Nutrient*	*Daily Need (%)*
Great	*Vitamin C*	176.3
	Vitamin B_9 (folate)	22.0
Good	*Vitamin B_5 (pantothenic acid)*	15.9
	Magnesium	15.0
	Manganese	13.0
	Potassium	9.8
	Phosphorous	8.3
	Dietary Fibres	8.0
Poor	*Vitamin B_6 (Pyridoxine)*	6.0
	Vitamin B_2 (riboflavin)	4.6
	Copper	4.2
	Vitamin B_1 (thiamine)	3.8
	Vitamin B_3 (niacin)	3.4
	Calcium	3.0
	Sodium, zinc, vitamin A equivalent, selenium, iron, vitamin E and vitamin K	Less than 3

There are a couple of caveats about the seed pods' nutrients, too.
- ✓ Raw seed pods contain a very high amount of vitamin C. But because they can only be consumed after cooking, some of the vitamin C gets destroyed. One study found that around 15 to 55 per cent of vitamin C can be lost in cooking.[9] Another indicated that depending on the cooking method, the loss could range from 10 to 100 per cent.[10] Microwaving, however, seemed to be the most effective option for retaining vitamin C. Although these studies did not specifically focus on cooking moringa, they provide a general idea about the temperature-dependent degradation of vitamin C.
- ✓ While moringa pods are full of fibre, most people do not ingest the entire drumstick. Instead, they typically chew it, extract the juicy flesh and discard the tough, fibrous skin. Consequently, they don't get much fibre. So, never blindly follow nutrition numbers without first asking yourself, 'Does this make sense? Could I be missing something?'

Moringa leaves and seeds contain many antioxidant and anti-inflammatory plant compounds.[11]
- ✓ **Quercetin:**[12] Exhibits antioxidant,[13] anti-inflammatory,[14] anti-allergic,[15] anti-cancer,[16] brain-protective[17] and heart-protective properties[18]
- ✓ **Kaempferol:** Antioxidant, anti-inflammatory, anti-cancer, antimicrobial properties. It also protects the heart, brain, bones, liver, lungs and digestive system.[19]
- ✓ **Myrecetin:** Antioxidant, anti-cancer and antimicrobial agent, and is known for its heart-protective and anti-diabetic properties.[20]

- ✓ **Chlorogenic acid:** Recognized for its liver-protective, anti-diabetic and anti-obesity attributes.[21]
- ✓ **Isothiocyanates:** Provide anti-cancer, anti-inflammatory, anti-microbial and neuroprotective benefits.[22]
- ✓ **Tannins:** Known for their anti-inflammatory, anti-cancer, heart-protective and liver-protective properties.[23]
- ✓ **Saponins:** Also offer anti-cancer benefits.[24]

It's therefore safe to infer that moringa leaves and seed pods possess similar health-enhancing properties.

HEALTH BENEFITS

Traditional Benefits

In Ayurveda, moringa leaves are considered helpful for combatting disorders caused by vata and kapha dosha imbalances. The leaves stimulate digestion and reduce intestinal parasites. The seed pods improve vision, clear complexion, cleanse the bladder and urinary tract, reduce abdominal problems, haemorrhoids and sleep disorders, increase breast milk production, lower obesity and swelling and increase strength. The seed pods are aphrodisiacs and improve semen quality. Moringa oil also helps treat wounds and skin diseases.[25]

Modern Benefits

Moringa has been found useful due to its antioxidant, anti-inflammatory, anti-diabetes, heart-protective and digestive benefits.[26]

Heart-Protective Benefits

✓ Moringa may help regulate blood cholesterol in the following ways:[27]
  1. It curbs the production of cholesterol.[28]
  2. It does not lower blood cholesterol below the normal levels.[29]
  3. Some of the cholesterol-lowering benefit is due to its antioxidant content.[30]
✓ Moringa targets anti-inflammatory compounds responsible for heart disease,[31] helping protect against heart disease.[32]
✓ Consuming moringa leaf extract regulates high blood pressure by relaxing the blood vessels and reducing oxidative stress.[33]
✓ It also amplifies the heart's ability to contract properly and prevents damage to delicate heart structures.[34]

Anti-Diabetic Properties

✓ Drinking moringa leaf extract can help prevent type 2 diabetes.[35]
✓ It can help improve blood glucose control among diabetics:[36]
  1. Some plant proteins in moringa leaves mimic insulin action and help reduce blood glucose.[37] This benefit is significant for diabetic people, who have insufficient insulin or insulin resistance (inability to help body cells use blood glucose), or both.
  2. It may aid in weight loss and reduce insulin resistance, problems observed in individuals with, or those who are developing, diabetes. These benefits are possibly due to the isothiocyanates in moringa.[38]

Anti-Cancer Benefits

- ✓ Moringa is known to be potent against many cancers.[39]
- ✓ It restricts the growth of pancreatic cancer cells in the body.[40] Typically, pancreatic cancer has an extremely poor survival rate because, with time, its cells become resistant to chemotherapy. The moringa leaf extract inhibits cell resistance to chemotherapy, improving its efficacy.[41]

Liver-Protective Benefits

Moringa may also protect against damage to the liver and kidneys,[42] probably due to the increased activity of antioxidant body enzymes when the extract is consumed.[43]

Joint-Protective Benefits

- ✓ It prevents joint destruction and soft tissue damage in rheumatoid arthritis.[44] This is due to the anti-inflammatory properties of the moringa extract.
- ✓ Even in traditional medicine, a paste of moringa leaf powder is applied to help relieve joint pain.

Bone-Protective Benefits

Moringa has been found to enhance bone density in laboratory animals.[45] This is believed to be due to the regulation of thyroid hormones. But please note, this result has yet to be observed in human trials.[46]

Digestive Benefits

- ✓ It may offer relief in various inflammatory digestive conditions such as ulcerative colitis, thanks to its anti-inflammatory compounds.[47]

- ✓ Moringa leaf extract has been found to protect against stomach and intestinal ulcers.[48]
- ✓ It can serve as a natural antimicrobial treatment for diarrhoea caused by certain types of bacteria.[49]

Neuro-Protective Benefits

The leaf extract may help safeguard against Alzheimer's disease by controlling some brain chemicals.[50]

Thyroid Benefits

Thyroid hormones regulate metabolism, which converts food nutrients into energy in the cells.[51] Although, there are varying claims about the benefits of moringa on the thyroid, here is the summary:

Thyroid function is governed by three main hormones: thyroid-stimulating hormone (TSH), secreted by a gland called the pituitary, which triggers the thyroid gland to produce two other hormones – triiodothyronine (T_3) and thyroxine (T_4). T_3 is the active hormone used by the body, while the latter must be converted into T_3 for use. The ultimate goal is to have normal T_3 levels.

An elevated TSH level suggests that the thyroid gland needs some stimulation to function correctly, a sign of an underactive thyroid or hypothyroidism.

Two scenarios can unfold: with the additional TSH stimulation, the thyroid gland can either produce enough T_3, or fail to generate sufficient amounts.

In the first scenario, where the thyroid functions adequately due to TSH stimulation, the diagnosis is subclinical hypothyroidism. The term 'subclinical' means that while the problem is present, there are no clinically visible symptoms because the T_3 levels are normal.

In the second case, where the thyroid gland fails to function despite TSH stimulation, leading to visible symptoms, the condition is referred to as clinical hypothyroidism.

- ✓ Research has shown that prolonged consumption of moringa causes hypothyroidism.[52]
- ✓ Similarly, moringa seems to reduce T_4 to T_3 conversion, which may potentially help patients with overactive thyroid or hyperthyroidism.[53]
- ✓ Newer studies suggest that moringa could improve thyroid hormone levels (increase T_3 and T_4, while decreasing TSH). So, it is believed to benefit patients with underactive thyroid or hypothyroidism[54], which contradicts the above.

It is worth noting that these were all animal studies. Until more information becomes available, if you suffer from thyroid problems, consume moringa in limited amounts, as provided later in the chapter.

HOW TO CONSUME

- ✓ All parts of the moringa tree can be consumed – leaves, bark, seed pods, pulp, roots and flowers. However, the bark, pulp and roots contain a toxic compound called spirochin that can cause paralysis and death when consumed in large quantities.[55] Thus, they are best avoided for direct consumption.
- ✓ The leaves can be eaten raw, steeped for tea or cooked in food preparation.
- ✓ They are dried and ground into powder before being sold as flour or capsules.

- ✓ Moringa leaves have a slightly bitter, grassy taste. They have a pungent flavour like horseradish. So, they go well with other dishes such as curries, dals, sambars and chutneys.
- ✓ They pair well with chillies, curries, tomatoes, potatoes, onions, shrimp, fish, chicken and coconut milk. They can be spiced up with garlic, ginger and turmeric.[56]
- ✓ Avoid overcooking moringa leaves to prevent them from becoming too bitter.
- ✓ In the Philippines, moringa leaves are steeped with lemongrass to make tea.
- ✓ Seed pods are eaten fresh – either roasted or cooked. They are highly fibrous on the outside, so the nutritious inner pulp is eaten, while the coarse exterior is discarded.
- ✓ Moringa seeds contain about 40 per cent oil, of a sweet, edible and non-sticking nature.[57] It is sometimes called ben oil due to its behenic acid contents.

HOW TO SELECT

- ✓ When buying, choose young, immature seed pods. Avoid those that are light coloured or soft, indicating age or spoilage.
- ✓ You can determine the seed pod's freshness by attempting to snap it. If the drumstick breaks in half, it is a young, tender and edible pod; otherwise, it might be old, fibrous and woody to taste. But don't offend the vendor by trying to bend and break all his produce!
- ✓ When buying a moringa oil bottle, it should look pale yellow in colour. Ensure the label explicitly confirms that the oil is for human consumption, as some moringa oil is also extracted for industrial, non-edible uses.

- ✓ Moringa powder should be rich green. A brown or even a pale green shade suggests it has low nutrition. Shade-drying moringa, instead of putting it out in the sunlight, preserves its green colour and nutrients.[58]

HOW TO STORE

- ✓ Do not wash moringa leaves unless you are ready to use them. Store them in a plastic bag in the refrigerator where they can last at least a week.
- ✓ Keep seed pods in an airtight container at room temperature.
- ✓ Moringa oil has a good shelf life of at least a year when stored in a refrigerator. It is one of the most stable oils, and does not turn rancid quickly. If unrefrigerated, it can be kept inside a dark glass bottle in a cool spot for up to six months.[59]

HOW MUCH TO CONSUME

- ✓ One can consume up to **3 cups** (**60 g**) of fresh moringa leaves daily.
- ✓ Since the leaves are about eighty per cent water, **3 tsp** (**12 g**) of dried leaf powder is equivalent to **60 g** of fresh leaves.
- ✓ You can consume **100 g** of fresh seed pods per day instead.
- ✓ Moringa leaf powder can help relieve oxidative stress in as little as 50 mg per kg of body weight.[59] So, an 80-kilogram person can get the required amount from **1 tsp** (**4 g**) of moringa powder daily. The higher amount indicated earlier is for better benefits.

- ✓ Research on animals suggests that a dose of 500 mg of moringa powder per kilogram of body weight can delay tumour cell growth. This is the equivalent of eating **10 tsp (40 g)** of moringa leaf powder a day for an 80-kilogram individual.[60] However, this is a substantial amount, which should not be consumed without medical supervision.
- ✓ For moringa tea, stir **1½ tsp (6 g)** of moringa powder in a cup (250 ml) of lukewarm water. Strain and discard the residue. It is best not to boil the mixture, as high temperatures can destroy some of the delicate antioxidant compounds in the powder.

HOW MUCH IS TOO MUCH

- ✓ No adverse effects have been seen when moringa is consumed in average food amounts.
- ✓ Intake beyond 12 g of moringa powder a day can raise the risk of getting loose motions.[61]
- ✓ Animal toxicity studies have shown that one gram of moringa powder per kilogram of body weight is safe.[62] This means an individual with an 80-kilogram body weight should not consume more than **20 tsp (80 g)** of powder a day to avoid toxicity.
- ✓ As of now, there are no studies on the toxicity levels of moringa seed pods.
- ✓ Taking all available data into account, it's advisable to draw the line at **200 g** of moringa leaves, **40 g** of moringa powder, or **300 g** of moringa seed pods daily. Do not exceed these quantities in one day.

WHO SHOULD AVOID

- ✓ People who have thyroid conditions – whether it's underactive or overactive – should refrain from consumption of moringa beyond standard dietary usage. No extra powder or tea, please!
- ✓ Pregnant and breastfeeding women should steer clear of moringa powder.[63] However, eating the leaves and seed pods as part of a balanced diet may be okay.
- ✓ If you take medicines for high blood pressure, do not overconsume moringa as it may lower the BP excessively.
- ✓ If you take diabetes medication, consuming too much moringa may lead to hypoglycaemia.

SUMMARY

Systems and Benefits	Major	Minor
Anti-inflammatory		■
Antioxidant		■
Bones		■
Brain		■
Cancer		■
Diabetes	■	
Digestive		■
Eyes		
Heart	■	
Immunity		■
Joints		■
Liver		■
Mental Health		
Pregnancy & Lactation		
Reproductive		
Respiratory		
Skin & Hair		■

Consumption: 3 cups (**60 g**) of leaves, **3 tsp** (**12 g**) of dried leaf powder or **100 g** of seed pods a day.

Excess: Do not exceed **200 g** of leaves, **40 g** of powder or **300 g** of seed pods daily.

19

SABJA
(SWEET BASIL SEEDS)
Fibre Friend

Ice was worth a fortune until about a century ago. Only the affluent could afford summer treats and drinks chilled with ice.

Roughly 2,500 years ago, the Persians, who ruled the region of modern-day Iran, mastered the art of ice storage. They harvested ice during the winter and kept it in expansive underground storage facilities topped with domes, known as a yakhchāl or 'ice pits'.

This ice remained available throughout the blistering heat of the desert summer, when it was used to prepare a luxurious dessert with honey, saffron and fruits.

As time passed, the recipe evolved: honey was replaced by sugarcane syrup, and rosewater was added to the mix. Eventually, delicate string noodles made from rice were combined with sweetened ice shavings. To balance the floral essence of the rose water, a splash of sharp lime juice was introduced. This slushy treat, topped off with crushed pistachios, was called faloodeh.

According to legend, Jahangir, son of Mughal emperor Akbar, was sent to conquer Iran. During this expedition, he encountered faloodeh and brought it back to India.

Today, this dessert is widely popular across the subcontinent, admixed with local garnishes, milk and ice cream. However, it is not complete without a dollop of sweet basil seeds, or sabja. This heavenly creation is now referred to as falooda, a fitting successor to the world's first ice cream.

Sabja seeds are derived from the sweet basil plant (scientific name *Ocimum basilicum*). This plant is recognized for its aromatic leaves, which are used as seasonings. Notably, sweet basil is distinct from holy basil, or tulsi (scientific name *Ocimum tenuiflorum*), indigenous to India. While the latter is employed in Ayurveda, courtesy of its medicinal properties, it is not a staple ingredient like sweet basil.

NUTRIENTS

The nutrient composition of sabja seeds varies depending on the region where they are grown.[1] Typically, they contain 10 per cent water, 60 per cent carbohydrates, 15 per cent proteins and 15 per cent fats. Of course, this is prior to being soaked in water.

Nutrition in Suggested Daily Amount of Sabja Seeds		Eat **15 grams**
		Has **66 calories**
Source	*Nutrient*	*Daily Need (%)*
Good	*Dietary Fibres*	8.5
	Manganese	7.6

Poor	*Magnesium, zinc, iron, vitamin A equivalent, vitamin B₁ (thiamine), vitamin B₂ (riboflavin), vitamin B₃ (niacin), Vitamin B₅ (pantothenic acid), vitamin B₆ (pyridoxine), vitamin B₉ (folate), vitamin C, vitamin E, vitamin K, calcium, copper, phosphorous, potassium, selenium and sodium*	Less than 3

✓ Various websites and some authoritative sources claim that sabja seeds contain numerous minerals such as calcium, iron, magnesium and zinc. However, these figures are based on the nutrient content per 100 g of dried seeds. Realistically, who would consume that much every day?

✓ Information about the nutrient profile of sabja is missing from many reputable international sources, likely because they are not prevalent in the developed western world. That has led to a variety of assertions from lesser-known industry sources. For instance, some claim that sabja seeds allegedly provide up to 11.5 per cent of our daily requirement for calcium. I had to dig deep into medical literature to check the veracity of such claims[1] – an effort most won't undertake. Effectively, the research shows that except for manganese, sabja doesn't provide any substantial quantities of vitamins or minerals. But they do contain the following plant nutrients:

1. **Alpha-Linolenic Acid (ALA):** This is an essential omega-3 oil, which has anti-inflammatory, anti-diabetes and heart-protective properties. It is beneficial against kidney disease, ulcerative colitis, rheumatoid arthritis, migraine headaches, depression, eczema,

psoriasis and respiratory conditions such as pneumonia and chronic obstructive pulmonary disease (COPD).[2] Approximately half the sabja fat content is ALA.[3] One tablespoon (15 g) of dry sabja seeds provides 1,250 mg of ALA, nearly fulfilling the daily requirement.
2. **Rosmarinic Acid:** This compound serves as an antioxidant, anti-inflammatory, anti-cancer, antimicrobial and antidepressant agent.[4]

HEALTH BENEFITS

Traditional Benefits

✓ Sabja seeds have been known to treat diarrhoea, indigestion, stomach ulcers, sore throat, fever and kidney disorders.
✓ They are renowned for their aphrodisiac and diuretic (eliminating water from the body) effects.
✓ Sabja seeds are used to treat chronic constipation and internal haemorrhoids.[5]

Modern Benefits

Sabja seeds are recognized for their antioxidant, anti-inflammatory, antimicrobial, anti-diabetic and heart-protective properties. They also possess digestive, anti-ulcer and anti-depressant properties.[6]

Antioxidant Benefits

✓ Sabja seeds can reduce free radicals and degenerative damage to various body parts.[7]

- ✓ Consuming them can reduce the risk of developing heart disease, brain-degenerative disorders, arthritis, diabetes and even certain cancers.

Anti-Inflammatory Benefits

- ✓ Sabja seeds help reduce body inflammation due to the anti-inflammatory omega-3 oil, ALA.[8]
- ✓ They may also help reduce inflammation due to the plant antioxidants within the seeds.

Digestive Benefits

Dry sabja seeds are tough to ingest and can be consumed only after being soaked in water for fifteen to thirty minutes. Since they are a significant source of dietary fibre, we will discuss this topic in more detail.

Dietary Fibres

They are called non-nutrients because the body cannot digest them. Most of their mass passes unused through the digestive tract. But they are critical to health; like water, with almost no nutrients yet essential for life.

Soluble and Insoluble Fibres

There are two types of dietary fibres: soluble and insoluble in water. A few are semi-soluble, which means they have properties from both types.
- ✓ Insoluble fibres increase the weight and volume of meals consumed. Softened and bulky food mass passes quickly through the intestines, preventing or easing constipation.[9]
- ✓ Constipation causes people to exert to defecate, resulting in haemorrhoids, which can be avoided or reduced by eating a high-fibre diet.

- ✓ People who don't eat enough fibre may develop diverticular disease that causes small pouches to form in the colon.[10] Diets high in fibre may protect against this disease.
- ✓ Soluble fibres slow the emptying of food from the digestive tract, prolonging satiety and helping reduce weight, body fat and waist-to-hip ratio.[11]
- ✓ Soluble fibres reduce the absorption of glucose[12] and cholesterol[13] in the intestines.
- ✓ Increased fibre intake is associated with improved immunity and lower incidences of type 2 diabetes, heart disease and stroke.[14]
- ✓ Soluble dietary fibres can help with diarrhoea or watery stools. People think that since fibre softens stools, it will worsen the symptoms of diarrhoea. However, the soluble fibres absorb excess water in the intestines and solidify the liquid bulk, relieving loose motions.
- ✓ Soluble fibres help constipation as they swell in contact with water to form a gel.[15] But they should be consumed with plenty of water; otherwise, they can aggravate constipation. In diarrhoeal situations, though, soluble fibres can be had without much water.
- ✓ While our bodies cannot digest dietary fibres, the helpful bacteria in our intestines can. Often, fibres are food for them. An adequate supply of such fibres maintains the bacterial health and prevents inflammation in the digestive tract, thereby protecting against inflammatory bowel disease.
- ✓ Dietary fibres reduce the risk of colorectal[16] and breast cancers.

So how much fibre should we eat daily?

Guidelines for Dietary Fibre Consumption

✓ The US Institutes of Medicine has issued the following fibre dietary recommendations:[17]

Age & Dietary Fibre	Men (g/day)	Women (g/day)
19–50	38	25
More than 50	30	21

✓ Americans typically eat 17 g of fibre daily.[18]
✓ The UK government guidelines are for 30 g of fibre per day, but most adults there eat about 20 g daily.[19]
✓ The Indian Council of Medical Research (ICMR) recommends **40 g** of dietary fibre a day for Indians.[20] Being a developing nation, processed foods are less common, so the fibre intake of Indians ranges from 15 to 41 g a day. But with growing availability of processed foods, which have fibres removed for better palatability, Indian urban dwellers should consider increasing their fibre intake.[21]

Sabja seeds offer 3.4 grams of dietary fibre a day, which is 8.5 per cent of our daily requirement. Our digestion is positively impacted by this superfood in a number of ways:

✓ Helps reduce glucose[22] and cholesterol[23] absorption in the intestines
✓ Contains pectin fibre that nurtures healthy intestinal bacteria, promoting their anti-inflammatory role[24]
✓ Sabja can alleviate constipation, diarrhoea and haemorrhoids (piles).

Weight-Loss Benefits

- ✓ Consuming the seeds can assist in combatting obesity.[25]
- ✓ Individuals who follow a calorie-restricted diet find it easy to stick to their diets when eating high-fibre meals.[26] This effect is due to increased satiety, delayed stomach emptying and reduced hunger pangs when on fibre-rich diets.
- ✓ Foods with water-soluble fibre, such as pectin, can enhance satiety, reduce calorie intake and lower body fat even on a high-fat diet.[27]

Anti-Diabetes Benefits

- ✓ Eating them can prevent sharp spikes in blood glucose levels after a meal.[28]
- ✓ Diets rich in water-insoluble fibres lower the risk of developing type 2 diabetes.
- ✓ Sabja seeds were found to control weight and blood glucose levels in a lab experiment.[29] Losing weight can help improve blood glucose control in people with type 2 diabetes.

Heart-Protective Benefits

- ✓ Sabja contains ALA, which reduces inflammation in the body, thereby protecting against heart disease.[30]
- ✓ The gel-like substance formed by water-soluble fibres in the intestines can inhibit cholesterol absorption.
- ✓ Increasing dietary fibre intake is associated with a reduced risk of dying from cardiovascular disease.

While there is little direct research on the heart-protective effects of sabja seeds, several experiments have been

conducted on basil oils, including holy basil (tulsi) oils. Those oils have been shown to:
- ✓ Reduce blood triglycerides and cholesterols.[31]
- ✓ Prevent these lipids from getting oxidised, which is a crucial step in heart disease progression.
- ✓ Reduce blood pressure and blood clotting tendencies.[32]

Since sweet basil and holy basil are different plants, drawing direct comparisons will not be accurate. Still, given their similar attributes, there is reason to be optimistic about the possibilities.

Anti-Cancer Benefits

- ✓ High-fibre foods reduce the risk of colon cancer.[33] This is because some dietary fibres are used as food by good bacteria in the intestines. As these fibres ferment, they produce healthy compounds called short-chain fatty acids, which have anti-cancer effects on colon cancer cells.
- ✓ While there are no studies on the effects of sabja seeds on colon cancer cells, what can we expect, given that sabja seeds are high in fermentable fibres?
- ✓ Lab experiments revealed that sabja seed extracts can cause the death of bone cancer cells.[34]
- ✓ Diets high in fibres reduce the risk of death from various types of cancers.

Immunity-Protective Benefits

Sabja seeds have antibacterial properties. They are effective against various bacteria, including the one that causes pneumonia.[35]

Of course, eating sabja is not a substitute for pneumonia treatment, which requires a doctor's consultation. But these findings can underscore the preventive benefits of regular sabja intake.

HOW TO CONSUME

Add a tablespoon of dry sabja seeds to a cup of water (one-fourth of a litre) for 15 to 30 minutes. In water, they start to release their digestive enzymes. As they absorb water, these black seeds develop a translucent, white-grey film, swelling to nearly triple their original size.

The soaked seeds by themselves are bland. You can incorporate them into shakes, smoothies or juices. If preferred, you can chew them in their swollen form.

HOW TO SELECT

Sabja seeds are easy to choose from the market, as long as they are food-grade quality and safe to eat.

Some enthusiasts like to harvest the seeds directly from sweet basil plants. But the gardening science behind it is detailed and beyond the scope of this book. For those interested, there are resources available.[36]

Sabja seeds are often confused with chia seeds. While the latter comes in a mix of white, grey and black, sabja seeds are jet black. Additionally, sabja seeds have an oblong shape, resembling a grain of rice, whereas chia seeds are oval. This book does not feature chia seeds because they are not endemic to the Indian subcontinent.

HOW TO STORE

- Sabja seeds are cheap and easily available at local markets. Buy them when you need. But if you want to store them long-term, they can last up to five years if kept in a dry, low-humidity environment.[37]
- Use a sealable plastic bag or glass jar for storage and place it in a cool, dark location.
- Once you soak the seeds in water, however, be cautious as pathogens can develop in the wet mixture. So, avoid keeping the soaked seeds out for too long.
- If you refrigerate soaked seeds, make sure to consume them within three to four days.

HOW MUCH TO CONSUME

Consume **1 tbsp (15 g)** of dry sabja seeds per day, after soaking them in water.

HOW MUCH IS TOO MUCH

Avoid consuming more than **1 tbsp** of dry sabja seeds a day.

WHO SHOULD AVOID

- If you are new to incorporating sabja seeds into your diet, slowly increase your consumption by ½ tsp (2.5 grams) every few days. Rapidly increasing dietary fibre intake is a sure way to cause stomach upset, bloating and, occasionally, loose motions.
- Sabja seeds are said to have a good concentration of

vitamin K, which helps in blood clotting. There is, however, no official source supporting this assertion. In fact, sabja seeds are said to increase blood-thinning action, not decrease – the latter would happen if they had high levels of vitamin K.

- ✓ If you are undergoing any elective surgery, don't consume sabja seeds two weeks before and after the surgery to prevent the risk of excess bleeding.
- ✓ Some argue that sabja lowers oestrogen and should be avoided during pregnancy. Also, since low oestrogen levels reduce female and male fertility, fertile couples who want to have children are advised to avoid them. While there is no research confirming that sabja lowers oestrogen levels, it might be better to exercise caution if you are pregnant or trying to have children.

SUMMARY

Systems and Benefits	Major	Minor
Anti-inflammatory		■
Antioxidant		■
Bones		
Brain		
Cancer		■
Diabetes	■	
Digestive	■	
Eyes		
Heart		■
Immunity		■
Joints		
Liver		
Mental Health		
Obesity	■	
Reproductive		
Respiratory		
Skin & Hair		

Consumption: 1 tbsp (**15 g**) of dry seeds daily, after soaking in a cup of water for fifteen to thirty minutes.

Excess: Don't consume more than **1 tbsp** a day.

20

BEETS
Endurance Booster

This is the story of how human greed and changing tastes reshaped our world.

Five hundred years ago, Europe fell in love with sugar. It commanded a high price as it was rare and exotic, categorized as both a spice and a medicine. As sugar consumption dramatically rose throughout Europe, a need for cost-effective mass production emerged to capitalize on this demand. Sugarcane, which thrived in flatlands near coastal waters – particularly where the soil colour was naturally yellow – was the ideal source. The perfect location for this was along the Atlantic coast of the Americas.

The European imperial powers set up sugarcane plantations in the Americas to transport sugar back to Europe.[1] To work the plantations, they enslaved millions of African individuals. This exploitation made sugar production inexpensive and subsequently contributed to a booming worldwide slave trade.[2]

Meanwhile, across the Atlantic in 1747, the chemist Andreas Marggraf introduced a method of producing sugar from beetroot,[3] which needs four times less water to grow than sugarcane. Since beets could be grown in Europe, local production of beet sugar became a financially viable alternative. Upon learning this, the king of Prussia, Frederick the Great, offered to subsidize beet sugar extraction. Subsequently, a sugar plant was established in Konari, Western Poland. By 1880, half of the world's sugar production shifted to beet sugar.[4]

As a result, the importance of the Americas in sugar production fell and with less money at stake, issues like slave emancipation gained recognition. One by one, countries in the Americas enacted laws against slavery, but this was less dictated by what the imperial powers thought of civil rights, and more influenced by the lowly beets reducing the profitability of American sugar trade.

So, when you consume beets next, remember its significant role in the abolition of slavery!

Beetroot is the tuber of the beet plant (scientific name *Beta vulgaris*). It originated in the Middle East and was cultivated by the ancient Egyptians and Greeks primarily for its green leaves. The Romans also utilized the plant for its roots. By the Middle Ages, people had started using beetroot to treat digestive and blood disorders.[5]

NUTRIENTS

Beets contain 88 per cent water, 9.6 per cent carbohydrates, 1.6 per cent proteins and 0.2 per cent fats.[6]

Nutrition in Suggested Daily Amount of Beets		Eat **200** grams
		Has **86** calories
Source	*Nutrient*	*Daily Need (%)*
Great	Vitamin B$_9$ (Folate)	109.0
	Manganese	32.9
Good	Magnesium	15.3
	Dietary Fibres	14.0
	Potassium	13.8
	Phosphorous	13.3
	Vitamin C	12.3
	Sodium	10.4
	Vitamin B$_6$ (pyridoxine)	6.7
	Vitamin B$_5$ (pantothenic acid)	6.2
	Iron	5.5
	Vitamin B$_2$ (riboflavin)	5.0
Poor	Vitamin B$_1$ (thiamine)	4.4
	Zinc	4.1
	Vitamin B$_3$ (niacin)	3.7
	Calcium	3.2
	Vitamin A equivalent, vitamin E, vitamin K, copper and selenium	Less than 3

Beets also contain many other beneficial plant compounds, such as:

- ✓ **Betalains:** Possess antioxidant, anti-inflammatory, anti-cancer and heart-protective properties.[7] These impart the red colour to beets.
- ✓ **Nitrates:** Reduce blood pressure, enhance blood flow and boost endurance.[8]

- ✓ **Polyphenols:** Protect against oxidative stress, inflammation, cancer and diabetes while also safeguarding the heart, brain, bones and the digestive system.[9]
- ✓ **Carotenoids:** While beet tubers contain no lutein or beta-carotenes,[10] they can be found in beet leaves.[11] Some sources highlight the presence of carotenoids in beets, while others don't.

Carotenoids offer various health benefits, including antioxidant, anti-inflammatory, anti-cancer and anti-diabetic properties, along with protecting the eyes, skin, heart, brain and the immune system.[12] However, to reap these benefits, you must cook and eat your beet leaves!

HEALTH BENEFITS

Beets have antioxidant, anti-inflammatory, anti-cancer, antimicrobial, heart-protective and brain-protective properties. They also offer digestive benefits and help improve endurance.[13]

Antioxidant and Anti-Inflammatory Benefits

- ✓ Betalains, polyphenols, nitrates and (in beet leaves) carotenoids offer many antioxidant benefits that prevent degenerative disorders.[14]
- ✓ Beets reduce inflammation in most organs of the body.[15]

Anti-Cancer Benefits

Betalains are the protective compounds responsible for this property of beets.[16] Few natural foods contain betalains, making beetroot a critical component of many anti-cancer diets. But the mechanism of its action still needs to be researched further.

Heart-Protective Benefits

- ✓ Help relax blood vessels and reduces systolic and diastolic blood pressures.[17] This could be due to their nitrates,[18] potassium[19] and vitamin B_9 contents[20].
- ✓ Protect against the oxidation of fats (called lipid peroxidation), a critical step in developing heart disease[21]
- ✓ Reduce the blood's clotting tendency, a risk factor for heart attacks or stroke[22]
- ✓ Dietary fibre in beets aids in reducing cholesterol absorption in the intestines, a feature useful for patients on cholesterol-lowering medicines.

Exercise-Related Benefits

For high-performance athletes, beets offer a fascinating mechanism by which their nitrates enhance endurance benefits.[23]

How Beets Help You Beat the Competition

- ✓ Beetroot juice provides nitrates that are absorbed into your blood and start circulating throughout the body, peaking within one to two hours after consumption.
- ✓ Nearly 25 per cent of these nitrates are quickly absorbed by the salivary glands and released in the saliva.[24] The glands cannot achieve this while you drink the juice, as they need the nitrates to be present in the blood for absorption.

- ✓ Some bacteria on your tongue convert the nitrates in the saliva into another set of compounds called nitrites.[25] So, beware if you tend to scrub your tongue hard after brushing every morning.
- ✓ What do you think happens if you use mouthwash after drinking beetroot juice? The nitrites in your saliva are significantly reduced.[26]
- ✓ As you swallow these nitrites through saliva, they are absorbed into your blood.[27]
- ✓ Within two to three hours of consuming beetroot juice, your blood nitrite levels also peak.[28] You must time this peak correctly.
- ✓ Certain blood proteins and enzymes convert the blood nitrites into the performance superstar: nitric oxide (NO), a compound that relaxes blood vessels and increases blood flow,[29] which is precisely what you need for breaking that world record!
- ✓ The icing on the cake are the two conditions that enhance this conversion of nitrites to nitric oxide – low blood oxygen and acidic blood pH.[30] When do you think a sportsperson encounters these conditions? It's when he is gasping for breath and his blood is flooded with lactic acid or lactate. In other words: during an all-out physical effort.[31]
- ✓ Blood nitrite levels gradually come down to normal levels over twenty-four hours.

I imagine a beetroot juice advertisement on the lines of a famous chewing gum one: 'We take care of your nitric oxide; the rest is up to you.'

Would you get the same benefit by eating beets instead of drinking beetroot juice? Certainly you could, but let's face it – which endurance athlete wants to eat half a kilogram of raw beets three hours before setting his personal best?

Here are some key points about beets:
- ✓ Drinking beet juice beforehand allows you to exercise longer.[32] It increases lung function and strengthens muscle contraction, which help improve cardiorespiratory endurance.[33]
- ✓ Consuming whole beets significantly improves running performance.[34] Athletes don't feel as exerted if they eat beetroot seventy-five minutes before the run. Of course, you might not run at your best while holding many beets in your belly. Please exercise discretion.
- ✓ Beetroot juice can improve cycling performance in trained cyclists.[35]
- ✓ How soon before activity should you consume beet juice? Three hours.[36] The levels of nitric oxide in the blood peak two to three hours after drinking the juice and return to normal within twelve hours.
- ✓ Older athletes and those who are not in the best shape appear to benefit the most from beet juice.[37]
- ✓ How much juice should you drink to take advantage of this benefit? Check the 'How Much to Consume' section later in this chapter.

Brain-Protective Benefits

- ✓ Beetroot nitrates can increase the blood flow to the brain, improving cognition (conscious thought, attention and memory).[38]
- ✓ Ageing individuals who exercised and drank beetroot juice experienced improved brain function similar to younger adults.[39]

✓ Type 2 diabetes patients showed faster reaction times after consuming beetroot juice.[40]

Joint-Protective Benefits

Beets are thought to decrease osteoarthritis discomfort by reducing joint inflammation.[41]

Digestive Benefits

✓ Beets have carminative (flatulence-relieving) properties.[42]
✓ Dietary fibre in beets promotes a healthy digestive system.
✓ Fibre may help prevent constipation and alleviate symptoms of inflammatory bowel disease (IBD).
✓ Dietary fibre also aids in reducing glucose absorption in the intestines, which is especially useful for type 2 diabetes patients.

HOW TO CONSUME

✓ Beets can be had raw in salads or cooked by steaming, boiling, frying and roasting. They make a great addition to soups, pasta and sauces and can even be fried into chips.
✓ Beet leaves can be eaten raw or sautéed.
✓ They can be juiced or added to smoothies.
✓ Beets pair well with spinach, kale, pears, raspberries and cheeses.[43]

HOW TO SELECT

There are three types of beets available in the market:

- ✓ **Red or purple beets:** The ones commonly associated with beetroot, their red colour comes from antioxidant and anti-inflammatory plant pigment compounds called betacyanins, a subset of betalain pigments. In most people, these compounds are digested, which changes their colour. However, in 10–14 per cent of the population,[44] the body cannot digest and break them down. So, they are absorbed in the blood and cleared through the kidneys or passed through the stools without absorption. As a result, individuals with this condition may experience pink or red urine (beeturia) or stools. While this is typically a benign condition with no cause for concern, if the sight of pink or red urine or stools is likely to spook you, it may be wise to monitor beet intake.
- ✓ **Yellow or golden beets:** Less sweet than the red varieties, they have a milder flavour. They are rich in other beneficial plant pigments called betaxanthins, a sub-group of betalain compounds, which are also beneficial but unlike their red brethren, they don't stain everything.
- ✓ **Chioggia beets:** These look red on the outside, but when sliced, reveal alternate stripes of red and white, an aesthetic enhancement to the salad bar. When cooked, all bands turn pale pink, making them best suited for raw consumption.

Note: Sugar beets used for sugar production are another type of beetroot, though they are not typically found in retail stores.

- ✓ Select tender and medium-sized beets, about two inches in diameter. Large ones are best avoided as they have a hard, woody core.
- ✓ Choose beets with intact skin.
- ✓ Soft ones should be avoided.
- ✓ Buy them a day or two before use, as they start losing nutrition over time, even with proper storage.
- ✓ If possible, buy beets with their green leaves still attached. Wilting greens are the first sign that the beets are not fresh. Without the greens, however, it is harder to assess their freshness.
- ✓ Raw beets are crunchy, and cooking turns them soft and creamy.

HOW TO STORE

- ✓ Cut off the greens about two inches above the beetroot before storing them, as the leaves will pull moisture out of the root otherwise. Avoid trimming too close to the top to prevent the purple juice from bleeding out.
- ✓ Beet greens can only survive for one to two days when stored within a plastic bag in the fridge.
- ✓ Without leaves, beetroot can last in the fridge for two to three weeks. If they are stored with the leaves, they will survive only a week in the refrigerator.
- ✓ Do not wash beets before refrigerating, as the excess moisture can rot them faster.
- ✓ Avoid keeping beets in plastic bags as the retained moisture will lead to condensation on the beet surface and faster spoilage.

- ✓ Store in a humid environment, such as the refrigerator's vegetable drawer. A closed drawer retains the moisture from the vegetable without making it too wet. Otherwise, the beets will dry out even in the fridge. You don't want too much moisture when storing beets, but dry air is not suitable either.
- ✓ Freezing beetroot is not a great idea, as they become mushy upon thawing.
- ✓ One option is to cook the beets before freezing. If wrapped properly in plastic, they can last up to nine months in the freezer.
- ✓ Fresh beetroot juice can be stored in the refrigerator for up to three days.

SHOULD YOU COOK BEETROOT?

Cooking beets reduces the absorption of their nitrates. It is also known to destroy some of the vitamin C in beets. On the other hand, there is an advantage: boiling reduces their oxalate content. Since oxalates reduce iron and calcium absorption and can cause kidney stones, cooking beets is not a bad idea either.

Ultimately, it comes down to personal choice, as cooked beets are creamier in taste.

HOW MUCH TO CONSUME

- ✓ Experts advise consuming about **1½ cups (200 g)** of beetroot a day. The recommendation is based on a daily intake of 800 mg of nitrates for an eighty-kilogram person.[45] Raw beets contain about 90 mg of nitrates

per hundred grams.[46] Since other foods will also supply nitrates, sticking to this amount will be prudent.
- ✓ One kilogram of beetroot will usually yield 600 ml of beetroot juice. So, consume **120 ml** of beetroot juice daily for the same nitrate benefit as above. Keep in mind that juicing removes dietary fibre, eliminating a significant source of health benefits.
- ✓ Cooking beets reduces the bioavailability of their nitrates. So, to gain their nitrate-related benefits, they are best consumed raw.
- ✓ For athletes, the best improvements are observed on consuming over 500 mg of nitrates at once. But this would require you to eat **550 g** of raw beetroot a few hours before an athletic event, a practical impossibility. The same results can be achieved with **330 ml** of beetroot juice. Some concentrated beetroot juices, which come in 70 ml 'shots', offer 400 mg per shot.[47] Taking two shots, the first three hours before the event and another two hours prior, can provide a significant nitrate boost.[48]

HOW MUCH IS TOO MUCH

It is advisable not to exceed the suggested amounts above because beets are high in oxalates that prevent the absorption of certain minerals.

WHO SHOULD AVOID

- ✓ People prone to developing kidney stones, as beet oxalates can increase the risk.

- ✓ Crimson urine and stools after eating beats can be harmless but alarming. If this concerns you, avoid beets.
- ✓ Pickled or canned beets often contain a high amount of sodium. If you are watching your blood pressure, rinse beets before eating.
- ✓ Inviduals on blood-pressure-lowering medicines, as the combined effect can lower the blood pressure excessively
- ✓ Pregnant women, as the nitrates may oxidize some of their haemoglobin and render it incapable of transporting oxygen – a condition called methaemoglobinaemia,[49] which can lead to headache, dizziness and fatigue. However, this condition is treatable and reversible.
- ✓ Breastfeeding women, as the effect of nitrates on infants below the age of one year is still not scientifically understood
- ✓ While some people think that consuming nitrates can generate cancer-causing compounds called nitrosamines in the body, the science behind this is more complex. Simply put, nitrates from vegetables are converted to nitric oxide in the body, which is beneficial. Whereas nitrates added for curing animal meats form nitrosamines.[50] So, beets are completely safe in this regard.

SUMMARY

Systems and Benefits	Major	Minor
Anti-inflammatory	■	
Antioxidant	■	
Bones		
Brain	■	
Cancer	■	
Diabetes		
Digestive		■
Eyes		
Heart	■	
Immunity		
Joints		■
Liver		
Mental Health		
Pregnancy & Lactation		
Reproductive		
Respiratory		
Sports-oriented	■	

Consumption: 1½ cups **(200 g)** of beetroot or **120 ml** of its juice daily. For sports performance, **330 ml** of juice three hours before the event.

Excess: Stay within the above levels.

APPENDIX A

WHEN IS A FOOD ITEM A GOOD NUTRIENT SOURCE?

'Which is a better source of dietary fibre: coconut flesh or coconut water?'

As we debate this question, we can determine if a food item is a good source of a nutrient, such as fibre in this case.

METHOD 1: EMPLOYING COMMON SENSE

Given that coconut meat is chewy and its water is a clear liquid, it's logical to assume that the former would be a better source of fibre. This is an example of making nutritional decisions using common sense. (Ironically, common sense is often said to be quite uncommon!) However, we would not have asked the question if the answer was so simple.

METHOD 2: USING A CHEAT SHEET

By referring to nutritional tables of coconut flesh and water in their chapter, we find that coconut flesh and coconut water provide 6.8 per cent and 6.9 per cent of our daily fibre needs, respectively. The latter wins by a tiny whisker. But how did that happen?

METHOD 3: THE ACCURATE BUT LABOUR-INTENSIVE PROCESS

A closer examination of the nutrient profiles of coconut meat[1] and its water[2] reveals that the two contain 9 g and 1.1 g of fibre for each. So, you were right; coconut flesh has eight times more dietary fibre than its water.

But look more closely. The above numbers are based on the consumption of a hundred grams per day. The advised amount is 30 g of coconut meat on a daily basis, giving you 2.7 g of fibre. Similarly, the suggested amount for coconut water is 250 ml daily. As 100 g of coconut water is nearly 100 ml since it is mostly water, a full glass (250 ml) will deliver 2.77 g of fibre, edging its solid rival by a coir-hair's breadth.

This detailed analysis may force you to ask:
- ✓ If the book had recommended drinking 240 ml of coconut water per day instead of 250 ml, would coconut meat be a better source of fibre than its water? Yes.

If that sounds illogical, remember that such calculations should always be based on each individual's health, unless you are writing a nutrition textbook, in which case you might only focus on the contents in 100 g of the food. For example, people with damaged kidneys may be advised to limit coconut water consumption to only 150 ml per day as their kidneys won't be able to flush out potassium as easily, leading to heart problems.[3] After all, people with moderate to severe kidney disease are told to restrict potassium intake to 3,000 mg a day instead of 4,700 mg, which is the upper recommended limit for people with healthy kidneys.[4]

In effect, for kidney disease patients, coconut flesh is a better fibre source than coconut water.

WHAT IS A GOOD SOURCE OF A NUTRIENT?

So, how do you decide if a food item is a good source of a specific nutrient?

The 5/20 Rule[5]

- ✓ A food that supplies more than **20 per cent** of the daily requirement of a nutrient is considered high in that nutrient and, hence, a **great** source.
- ✓ One that contains less than **5 per cent** of the daily requirement is deemed to have a low nutrient content and is typically viewed as a **poor** source.
- ✓ When a food provides between **5** and **20 per cent** of the daily nutrient requirement, we're in a grey area, an in-between land. We can choose to call it a **good** source in this case.

Applying this rule allows us to determine, based on the tables in each chapter, whether a food item is a good source of certain vitamins and minerals. But what exactly constitutes these daily requirements? For this, we use something known as the 'Daily Value'.

DAILY VALUE (DV)

Different health organizations propose a recommended dietary allowance (RDA) for nutrients. These are the amounts that should be consumed daily to prevent deficiencies and are calculated based on scientific research. However, for some nutrients, such values may still be unknown. So, health experts propose a daily value (DV), which is similar to RDA but with less scientific backing. Therefore:

- ✓ When RDA is known, DV is RDA.
- ✓ When RDA is unknown, a reasonable DV is suggested by the experts.

DV values can vary marginally from country to country. In this book, we've used the values recommended by the Indian government.[6] And we've limited our considerations to adults, both men and women, under fifty years of age. We also chose the larger of the two numbers if the DVs differed for men and women. For example:

- ✓ For iron, women are told to take 29 mg versus 19 mg for men a day
- ✓ For vitamin A, men are advised 1,000 µg as against 840 µg for women daily

We've consequently used 29 mg and 1,000 µg for iron and vitamin A, respectively, for our calculations. If an Indian guideline is absent for a certain nutrient, we refer to the nutrient recommendations provided by the US National Institute of Health.[7]

Appendix C features a summary table showcasing nutritional content of the twenty Indian superfoods featured in this book and their corresponding DVs. This will also identify which foods are poor, good or excellent sources of various nutrients.

WHAT HAPPENS IF WE INCREASE INTAKE?

Here's another common query: What if we were to increase our food intake two-fold? Take carrots, for example; they are considered a poor source of magnesium since the recommended quantity of 100 g only delivers 4 per cent of the daily requirement. But what if one were to consume 200 g of carrots a day? This would cater to 8 per cent of the nutrient requirement, thereby categorizing carrots as a good source. Should one decide to ingest half a kilogram of carrots daily – a horrendous thought – it would undoubtedly serve as an excellent magnesium source. However, one must be then ready for the often-unsavoury repercussions of exceeding the stipulated consumption quantity.

Welcome to the naïve world of food nutrition, where it is so simple to tweak conclusions to suit your narrative, product and service offerings.

BEWARE OF ONLINE MISINFORMATION

Consider a scenario where you're curious to know if onions are a good source of vitamin B_9. Your first instinct might be to search the internet. But, please keep in mind the following advice before doing so:
✓ The internet is rife with misinformation, whether intentional or not.

- ✓ Many websites are nothing more than well-curated compilations of information lifted from elsewhere.
- ✓ Even though artificial intelligence (AI) is used to enhance online information, current AI technologies still can't distinguish between fact and fiction. Their goal is mainly to gather and reformat existing data.

> 'Beware of false knowledge; it is more dangerous than ignorance'
> – GEORGE BERNARD SHAW, Irish playwright and critic

As a result, you are likely to see the same incorrect information circulating and possibly reinforcing beliefs, such as 'Cinnamon is a great source of calcium, iron, zinc and magnesium.' You might consume your cinnamon latte for years, hoping for stronger bones and boosted immunity, only to find no discernible improvement in your health!

The following guide can save you a lot of confusion and potential health complications from years of misguided consumption.

HOW TO DETERMINE IF A FOOD ITEM IS A GOOD SOURCE OF A NUTRIENT?

This section is slightly technical, which is why it is provided in an appendix – feel free to skip if it does not interest you.

Step 1: Consult Authority Websites

Look for government websites, such as the US Department of Agriculture,[8] Australian Food Composition Database

Search[9] or Centre for Food Safety (Government of the Hong Kong Special Administrative Region)[10]. Some other examples include the WebMD Ingredients Guide[11] or, at times, Wikipedia,[12] but be more alert when using non-government websites.

Also, exercise caution while perusing nutritional information on websites promoting their own 'specially formulated' products or services. Such websites may exaggerate minor benefits based on flimsy or baseless evidence.

Step 2. Verify the Correct Fruit or Vegetable

Let's say you want to know if sabja is rich in magnesium. If you search for 'iron in basil seeds', you will find that it has 15.1 mg of iron per 100 g.[13] Consuming an average daily amount of 15 g gives approximately 8 per cent of your daily iron requirements, making sabja seem like a good source of iron. But hold on! Sabja is typically referred to as 'sweet basil' in English (scientific name *Ocimum basilicum*), which is frequently confused with tulsi or 'holy basil' (scientific name *Ocimum tenuiflorum*). Both plants produce seeds, and many websites carelessly refer to tulsi as basil. Sweet basil (sabja) seeds contain only 2.3 mg of iron per 100 g, almost seven times less than tulsi seeds. Consequently, sabja only provides about 1 per cent of your daily iron requirement, making it a poor iron source. It would have been more accurate to search for 'iron in sweet basil seeds' rather than 'iron in basil seeds.'

Adding to the complexity, sweet basil has many varieties, including cinnamon basil and dark opal basil, with the most common being anise or persian basil. You should, therefore, search for *Ocimum basilicum* 'Liquorice' or '*Ocimum basilicum L*'[14].

Different types of papaya (such as Mexican, Hawaiian and Bangkok) have varying nutritional profiles. When websites like the US Department of Agriculture provide nutrient information on papaya, they often don't specify which variety they're referring to.[15] Sometimes, the data can be an average derived from multiple studies.

As we pointed out in the papaya chapter, the nutrient content of a fruit changes as it ripens, so it's unrealistic to expect precise beta-carotene content. Unlike the fixed specifications of your car engine, the lycopene content in your tomatoes won't be exact.

Step 3. Check Alternate Names for the Ingredient

In India, bell peppers are called capsicum. However, in the US, 'capsicum' typically refers to chilli peppers like cayenne and jalapeño, which are hot and spicy despite sharing the same scientific name, *Capsicum annuum*. Consequently, when American websites mention the vitamin and mineral contents of 'capsicum', they're referring to chilli peppers. This confusion can also make it quite difficult to deduce which variety is being discussed on an Indian website unless it's explicitly stated.

Step 4. Consider the Part of the Plant being Consumed

Coconut flesh and coconut water have significantly different nutrient profiles. The same applies to pineapple fruit and juice; or moringa leaves and seed pods.

Step 5. Determine Nutrient Amount Based on Your Typical Consumption Quantities

Official websites provide the nutrient contents of a fruit or vegetable per 100 g to standardize information. But many of them neglect to consider whether people typically consume 100 g of a particular food daily. For example, garlic, is touted to be an excellent source of vitamin B_6 (95 per cent DV) and manganese (80 per cent DV) on some websites.[16]

So, these proportions only hold if you're consuming 100 g of garlic daily – an impossibly large and harmful amount. When you adjust the daily consumption to a more reasonable 4 g, garlic's vitamin and mineral contents are practically negligible.

Step 6. Check Your Country's RDAs or DVs

Different countries propose varying amounts of daily nutritional intake, based partly on genetic variation or prevalence of certain illnesses. For instance, people of Indian or Chinese descent may require different vitamin A or phosphorous amounts daily compared to Americans.[17] Practicality, government reluctance or vested interests can also result in differences in guided numbers. These suggested amounts are also periodically revised based on new data.

Step 7. Consider Unique Factors like Age Group, Gender and Life Stage

The DV numbers change based on gender, ethnicity, age group and life stages, such as pregnancy or post-menopause.

Use the specific numbers applicable to your circumstances for accurate calculations.

These seven steps require some effort, and the appendix C of this book attempts to simplify the process for these twenty ingredients.

Step 8. Consider How Food is Processed

Just because a vegetable contains certain nutrients does not mean they will end up in your body. Remember that cooking food destroys 15 to 30 per cent of vitamin C. So, if you eat cooked bell peppers, your vitamin C intake will be lower than you might expect.

On the other hand, cooking is also known to help release certain nutrients from their tough fibrous matrices. For example, the antioxidant activity of tomatoes increases by 30 to 60 per cent on cooking, as its bound lycopene is released.[18] Tomato ketchup offers five times more lycopene than raw tomatoes. Therefore, if you don't mind raised eyebrows, skip your tomato salad and slurp the purée to get a tenfold bump in your lycopene intake.

Step 9. Understand Absorption, Synergy, Anti-Nutrients and Other Factors

Just because a nutrient enters your body does not mean you will be able to absorb all of it. Consider this analogy: if I give you a piece of chocolate, you may merrily gobble it. But what if I share ten? Most likely, you will stop after the fifth or the sixth piece. So, while you got ten chocolates, your body only got six.

Similar things happen within the body. If I give you just one microgram of vitamin B_{12}, your body will absorb nearly 60 per cent of it. But if you take 1,000 μg in one go, your body will wisely absorb only 0.5 per cent at best. What you do to chocolates, your body does for vitamin B_{12}.

Additionally, some nutrients help or compete with each other for absorption. For example, vitamin C increases iron absorption.[19] This effect is seen with iron in plant foods, such as chickpeas, figs and raisins. And vitamin C does not affect iron absorption from animal foods such as poultry.

Conversely, drinking tea, coffee or wine reduces iron absorption.[20] Confusingly, this effect of coffee is not drastically different across iron sources: one trial found that caffeine may reduce iron absorption from vegetarian sources by 64 per cent and non-vegetarian sources by 39 per cent.[21]

Numerous combinations of vitamins and minerals like this exist in nature.[22] It may be worth remembering them only if you plan to appear for a nutrition-related examination. But do note two key points:

- ✓ Vitamins A, D, E and K are fat-soluble and are better absorbed with some fats. Foods high in these vitamins should be consumed with your meals.
- ✓ Various B vitamins and vitamin C are water-soluble and don't need fats for absorption.

Additionally, you need to be aware of anti-nutrients. While spinach is rich in iron and calcium, our body cannot absorb 95 per cent of them because the oxalates bind tightly to both iron and calcium, preventing their absorption in the intestines. Anti-nutrients like oxalates can significantly reduce the number of nutrients absorbed by the body.[23]

Step 10. Be Mindful of Plant-to-Plant Variations

Despite taking the precautions stated above, we must note that food items are notorious for their diversity. You will get different amounts of nutrients in the same plant depending on the soil quality, temperature and region. Harvesting the same vegetable at various stages of its development will also yield varying nutrient profiles.

KEY TAKEAWAY

By now, hopefully, this book has managed to successfully explain why food-based nutrient trials will never provide definitive answers in the same way that chemical-based medicinal trials do. This is probably the most important message of this book.

Over the last twenty-five years of my career in preventive health, I have come across hundreds of highly educated people with ill-conceived ideas about biostatistical superiority of double-blind, placebo-controlled pharmaceutical trials, demanding the same rigour from food nutrients.

Even if this sounds harsh, don't allow your formal education to override common sense. Nutrients, such as vitamin A, can enter your body via a variety of routes, whereas medications, for example, atorvastatin, have only one. Your reading of this book indicates that your ancestors consumed nutrients similar to the former and lived sufficiently long; so, there shouldn't be any need for additional evidence to support these nutrients' contribution to your health. Further, this book is certainly not suggesting that anyone discontinues their medical treatment to rely solely on these superfoods as a cure; you should eat them for better health, and if it improves your medical condition, all the better. Modern interventions like atorvastatin, on the other hand, must prove their worth beyond a doubt; they have only one reason for being in your body, and that purpose must be rigorously verified.

In other words, the choice to consume carrots should not hinge on whether scientists can conclusively prove their benefits for eye health. We should incorporate them into our diets regardless, given their longstanding safe use by our ancestors. Any decision to avoid them should stem from research demonstrating the harm caused by their consumption.

In this way, superfoods necessitate an approach to health and wellness that stands in stark contrast to that of medicines..

APPENDIX B

SUMMARY OF HEALTH BENEFITS FROM NUTRIENTS

Benefits \ Food Item	Aloe Vera	Amla	Asafoetida	Beets	Capsicum	Carrots	Cinnamon
Anti-inflammatory	■	■	□	■	□	□	■
Antioxidant	■	■	□	■	■	■	■
Bones						□	□
Brain		□	□	■			□
Cancer	□	■	□	■	■	□	□
Diabetes	■				■		■
Digestive	■	■	■	□		□	□
Eyes		□			■	■	
Heart		■	□	■	■	□	■
Immunity	□	■	□			□	■
Joints				□			
Liver		□	□				□
Mental Health			□				
Pregnancy & Lactation						□	
Reproductive			■			□	
Respiratory			□				
Skin & Hair	■	■				■	■

■ Major Benefit   □ Minor Benefit

Coconut	Flaxseeds	Garlic	Ginger	Green Tea	Jamun	Moringa	Papaya	Pineapple	Sabja	Spinach	Tomato	Turmeric
	■	■	■	■	□	□	■	■	□	□	■	■
	□	■	■	■	■	□	■		□	■	■	■
	□	□		□		□				■	□	
■	□	□	□	■		□					□	■
	■	■	■	□	□	□	■	□	□	□	□	■
	□	□	■	□	■	■	□			■	□	□
	■	□	■		■	□	■	■	■	□		■
								■			■	□
	■	■	■	■	■	■	■	□	□	■	■	■
□	□	■	□		□	□	■	□	□		□	■
	□	□	□	□		□	□	■			□	□
		□				□						■
				□								□
			□						■	□	□	
												□
					□		□				□	□
■	□					□		□		□	□	■

APPENDIX C

OVERVIEW OF NUTRIENTS IN FOOD ITEMS

☐ Less than 5 per cent   ☐ 5 per cent to Less than 20 per cent

Benefits / Food Item	Units	Daily Value	Aloe Vera	Amla	Asafoetida	Beets	Capsicum	Carrots	Cinnamon	Coconut Meat
Daily consumption	g or ml		80	100	0.5	200	150	100	4	30
Calories	cal	2000	12	48	1.4	86	41	41	10	106
Dietary Fibre	g	40	0	5	0	5.6	2.7	2.8	2.1	2.7
Vitamin A, equivalent	µg	1000	0	97	0	4	236	835	1	0
Vitamin B$_1$ (thiamine)	mg	1.4	0	0.03	0	0.06	0.08	0.07	0	0.02
Vitamin B$_2$ (riboflavin)	mg	1.6	0	0.01	0	0.08	0.21	0.06	0	0.01
Vitamin B$_3$ (niacin)	mg	18	0	0.2	0	0.7	1.5	1.0	0.1	0.2
Vitamin B$_5$ (pantothenic acid)	mg	5	0	0.3	0	0.31	0.48	0.27	0	0.09
Vitamin B$_6$ (pyridoxine)	mg	2	0	0.1	0	0.13	0.45	0.14	0.01	0.02
Vitamin B$_9$ (folate)	µg	200	0	6	0	218	71	19	0	8
Vitamin C	mg	80	3	478	0	9.8	213	5.9	0.2	1.0
Vitamin E	mg	10	0	0.16	0	0	2.37	0.68	0.09	0.07
Vitamin K	µg	55	0		0	0	11.1	13.2	1.2	0.1
Calcium	mg	1000	6	25	3	32	9	33	40	4
Copper	mg	2	0	0.1	0	0	0.06	0.05	0.01	0.13
Iron	mg	29	0.1	0.9	0.2	1.6	0.5	0.3	0.3	0.7
Magnesium	mg	300	0	10	0	46	17	12	2	10
Manganese	mg	2	0	0.1	0.01	0.66	0.18	0.14	0.7	0.45
Phosphorous	mg	600	0	21	0	80	41	35	3	34
Potassium	mg	4700	0	198	0	650	320	320	17	107
Selenium	µg	40	0	0.6	0	0	3.8	0.1	0.1	3
Sodium	mg	1500	6	13	0	156	5	69	0	6
Zinc	mg	17	0	0.12	0	0.7	0.3	0.24	0.07	0.33

▫ 20 per cent or More

Coconut Water	Flaxseeds	Garlic	Ginger	Green Tea	Jamun	Moringa Leaf	Moringa Pods	Papaya	Pineapple Fruit	Pineapple Juice	Sabja	Spinach	Tomato	Turmeric
250	15	6	4	750	100	60	100	150	165	250	15	75	100	6
48	80	6	3	7	60	36	37	65	83	150	66	17	18	19
2.8	4.1	0.1	0.1	0	1.7	1.2	3.2	2.3	2.3	2	3.4	1.7	1.2	1.4
0	0	0	0	0	1	227	22	71	5	5	0	352	42	0
0.08	0.25	0.01	0	0.05	0.01	0.15	0.05	0.03	0.13	0.24	0	0.06	0.04	0
0.14	0.02	0	0	0.45	0.01	0.40	0.07	0.04	0.05	0.05	0	0.14	0.02	0.01
0.2	0.5	0	0	0.2	0.3	1.3	0.6	0.5	0.8	0.7	0	0.5	0.6	0.1
0.11	0.15	0.02	0.01	0	0	0.08	0.79	0.29	0.35	0.25	0	0.05	0.09	0.03
0.08	0.07	0.05	0.01	0.03	0.04	0.72	0.12	0.06	0.18	0.19	0	0.15	0.08	0.01
8	13	0	0	0	0	24	44	57	30	13	0	146	15	1
6	0.1	1.2	0.2	2.3	14.3	31	141	93	78.9	23.8	0	21	14	0
0	0.05	0	0.01	0	0	0	0	0.45	0.03	0.03	0	1.52	0.54	0.27
0	0.6	0.1	0	0	0	0	0	3.9	1.2	0.8	0	362	7.9	0.8
60	38	7	1	0	19	111	30	54	21	35	0	74	10	10
0.1	0.18	0.01	0.01	0.03	0	0.06	0.08	0.07	0.18	0.22	0	0.10	0.06	0.08
0.7	0.9	0.1	0	0.2	0.2	2.4	0.4	0.8	0.5	0.7	0.3	2	0.3	3.3
63	59	1	2	8	15	88	45	32	20	35	5	59	11	12
0.36	0.37	0.07	0.01	1.38	0	0.22	0.26	0.06	1.53	2.8	0.15	0.67	0.11	1.19
50	96	6	1	0	17	67	50	29	13	15	0	37	24	18
625	122	16	17	60	79	202	461	91	180	305	0	419	237	125
2.5	3.8	0.6	0	0	0	0.5	0.7	0.9	0.2	1	0	0.8	0	0.4
263	5	1	1	8	14	5	42	12	2	3	0	59	5	2
0.25	0.65	0.05	0.01	0.08	0	0.36	0.45	0.12	0.20	0.25	0.24	0.4	0.17	0.27

NOTES AND REFERENCES

To view the notes and references, scan the QR code provided below. Since this text contains over 1,600 references, they have been listed on a website rather than being appended to the main body of the book.

Most notes also include a link that allows you to read the original paper or document from which a particular section has drawn information.

The webpage is hosted on the author's website. To view the notes and references, scan the QR code provided below or visit the following link: https://healthsachet.com/superfoods-refs/.